40 Intense Parallel Bar Dips for Maximum Cut & Definition

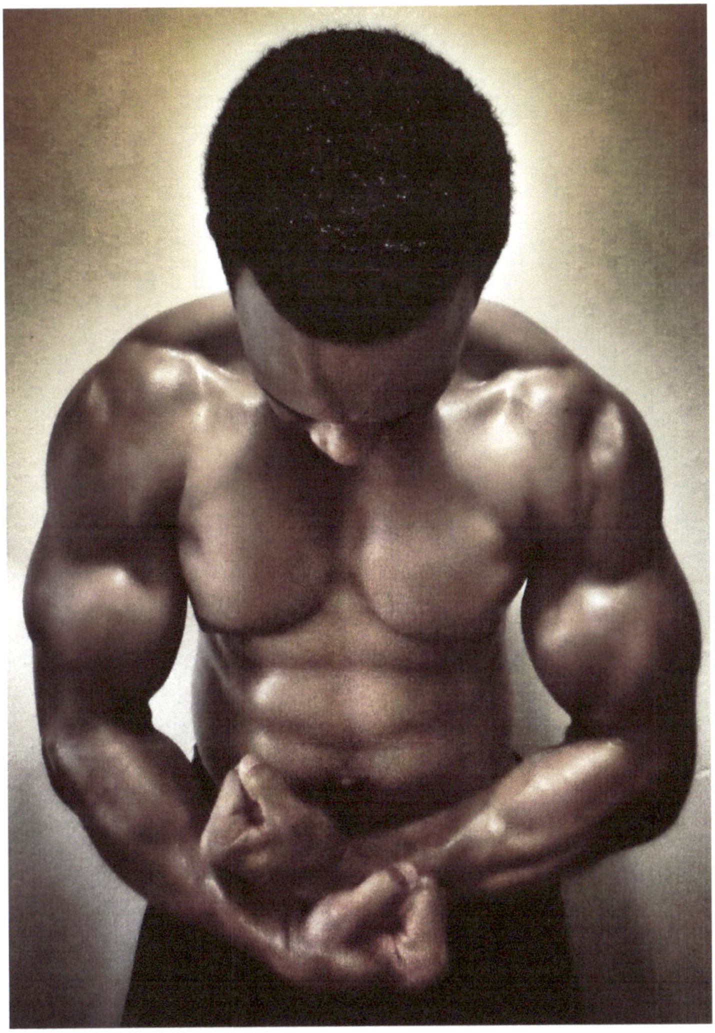

First Printing, 2016

ISBN 1-5196914-8-3

Acknowledgments

First and foremost, I'd like to give ALL the honor, glory, and praise to my Lord and Savior Jesus Christ for blessing and empowering me with the wisdom, revelation knowledge, understanding, and the physical commitment gift and drive to write this workout book. Your Precious Holy Spirit continues to lead, guide, and teach me how to walk by faith and not by sight, despite all the persecutions from the world. Once again I say thank you Jesus Christ. (Matthew 6:33, Philippians 4:13, 2 Corinthians 5:7)

Secondly, I want to thank my loving, virtuous wife, Charlene, for her endless love and continued support to encourage and drive me to write this workout book. None of this is possible without her and her love.

And to my two boys who think I am superman, Joshua and Caleb. Daddy loves you!

Table of Contents

Introduction – The Purpose of the Parallel Bar Exercise

When someone thinks of the parallel bars, usually the first thing that comes to mind are gymnasts. But this classic piece of gymnast equipment shouldn't be limited to just the professionals. Parallel bars are a great addition to your workout program for all people ages, shapes and sizes. There are so many exercises you can perform with these bars from beginners to the most advanced athletes in the world.

If you are a beginner, it's wise to have a workout partner with you to help spot each other. Another helpful key as a beginner is to use a padded floor or mats especially if you're trying a new skill or exercise for the first time. Remember, safety and perfect form is vital and foremost.

These exercises will also work your body from head to toe depending on your level of fitness. Additionally, parallel bars are great for people recovering from various injuries, debilitation conditions, and some illnesses. This is why they are highly used in rehabilitation centers and physical therapy offices.

Here are 10 advantages to using parallel bars:

1. Increase body weight strength
2. Allows for a more deeper range of motion
3. Increases body weight balance and coordination
4. Increases abdominal strength
5. Increases muscle endurance and stamina
6. Helps develop serious definition
7. Helps reduces body fat
8. Increases your athletic ability
9. Helps strengthen hand balance
10. Increases and develops body weight stabilization

In this book I've put together 40 different exercises performed on the Barbarian Parallel Bars. These particular bars are for the more advanced workout enthusiast. Because unlike traditional parallel bars that are attached to the floor in the gym or cemented in the ground at the park, the Barbarian Parallel Bars requires the individual to control the balance of the bars. This will cause your core to be increasingly engaged and will help take your strength and fitness level to an all-time high.

These workouts will cover you from the beginner main-move dip exercise to 39 of the most creative variation movements ever seen on a set of parallel bars. So whether you're a professional gymnasts, bar athlete at the park, or just simply a calisthenics body weight enthusiast, you can't go wrong by using and adding these bars to your weekly training program.

Welcome To the Exercises

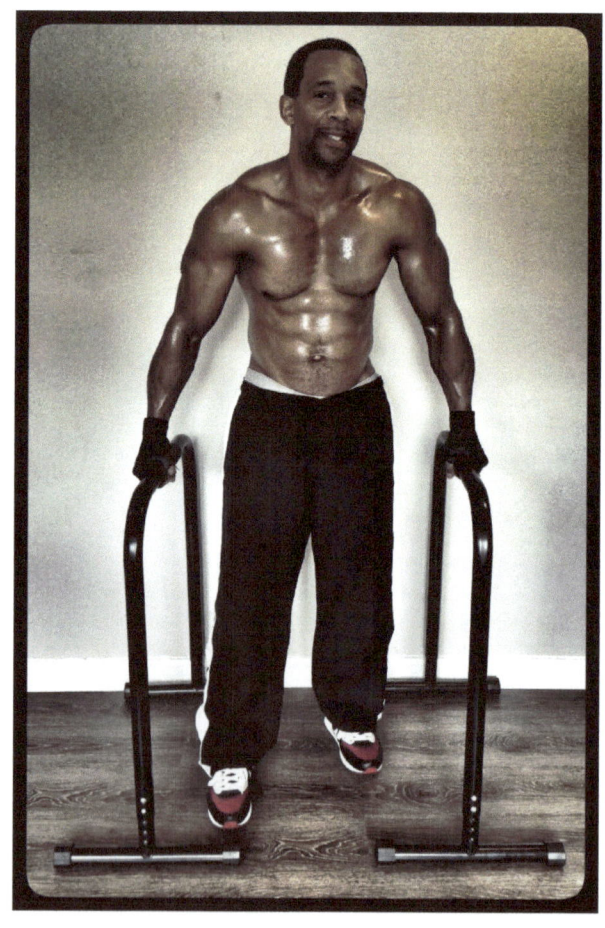

Chapter 1
Dips: Powerful Ripped Triceps

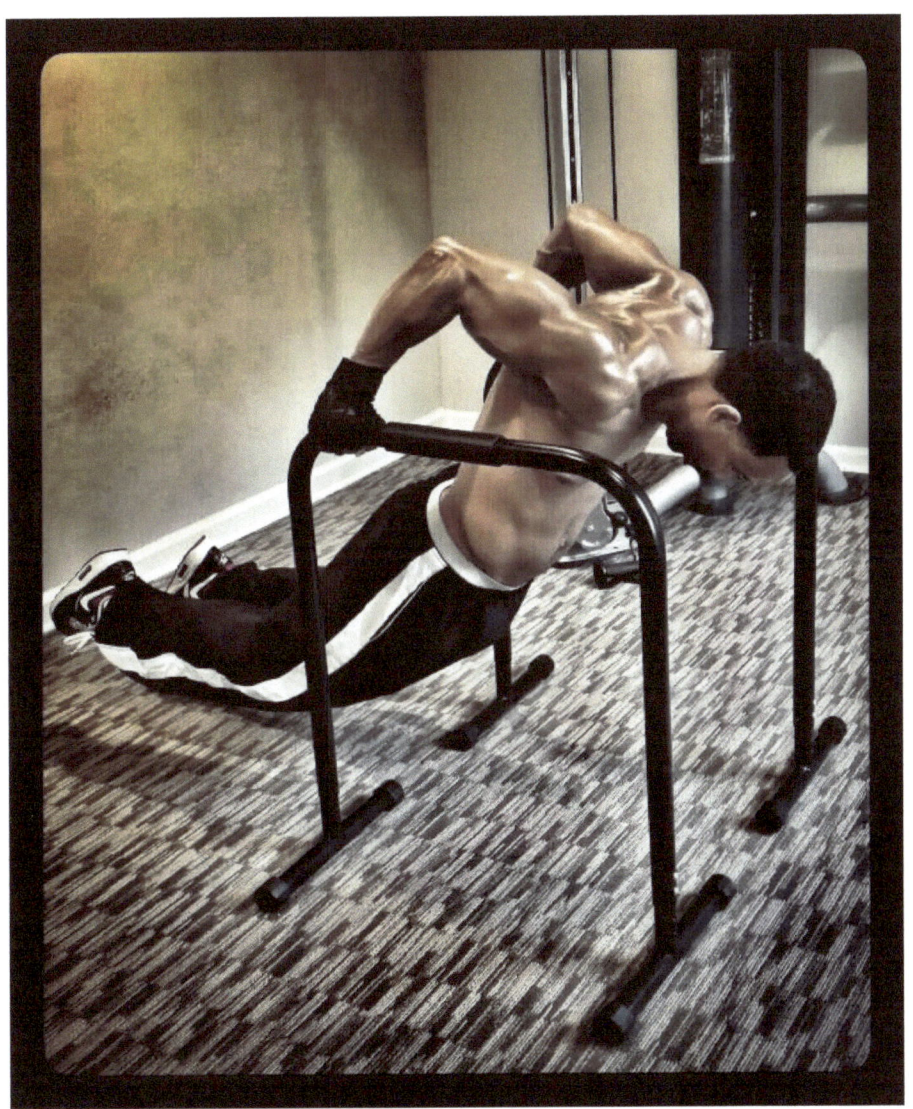

Main Move

Variation #1 - Dips
Muscles Worked: Triceps, Chest, Abdominals

How to:

1. Elevate your body up on the parallel bars with your arms fully extended and your legs bent back behind you. (Do not cross your feet). This is your starting position.

2. Engage your core and slowly lower your body down while breathing in. Keep your body in control without swinging. Pause for a second at the bottom.

3. While breathing out, raise your body back up to the starting position.

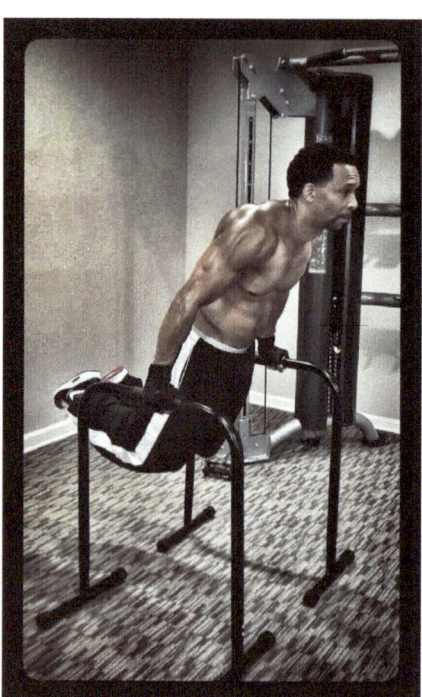 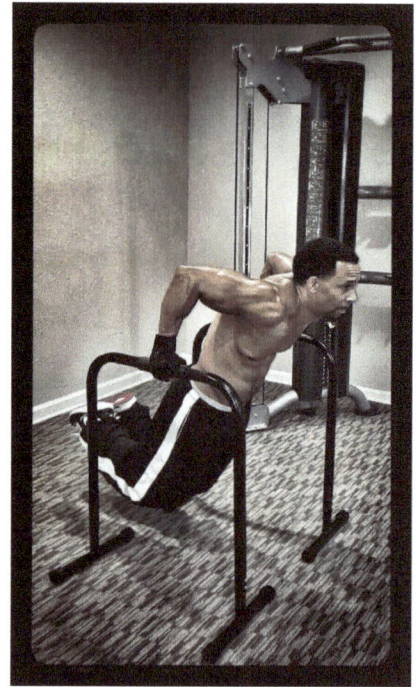

Variation #2

<u>Leaning Dips</u>
Muscles Worked: Triceps, Chest, Shoulders, Abdominals

How to:
1. Elevate your body up on the parallel bars with your arms fully extended, but this time tilt your body forward with your legs fully extended down. This is your starting position.

2. Engage your core and slowly lower your body down while breathing in. Keep your body tilted forward without swinging. Pause for a second at the bottom.

3. While breathing out, raise your body back up to the starting positon.

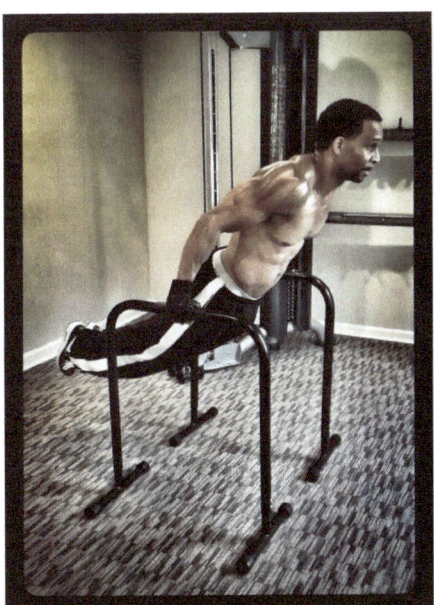 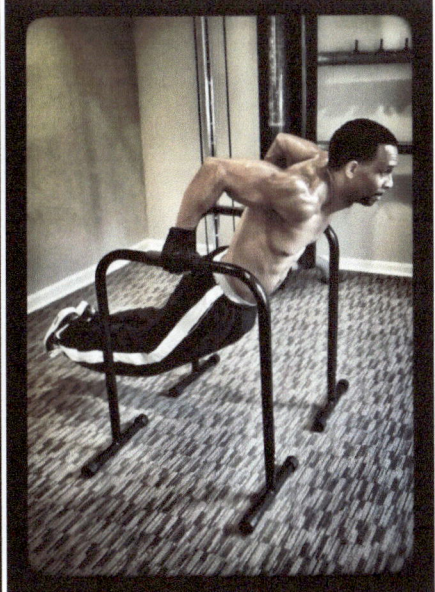

Variation #3
<u>Extra Deep Dips</u>
Muscles Worked: Triceps, Chest, Shoulders, Upper Back, & Abdominals

How to:
1. Elevate your body up on the edge of the parallel bars with your arms fully extended and your body tilted forward with your legs fully extended down.   This is your starting positon.

2. Engage your core and slowly lower your body down with your legs slightly bent until your shoulders are stretched past the 90 degree angle. Breathe in and pause for a second at the bottom.

3. While breathing out, raise your body back up to the starting position.

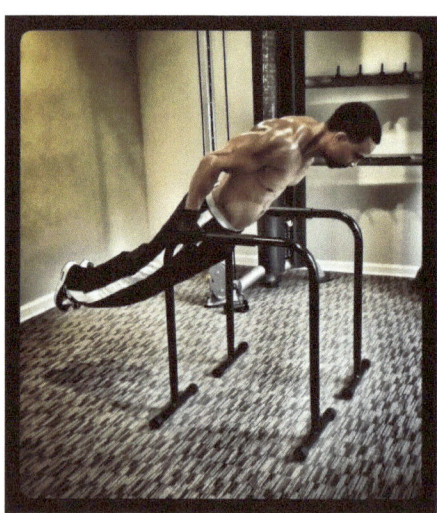 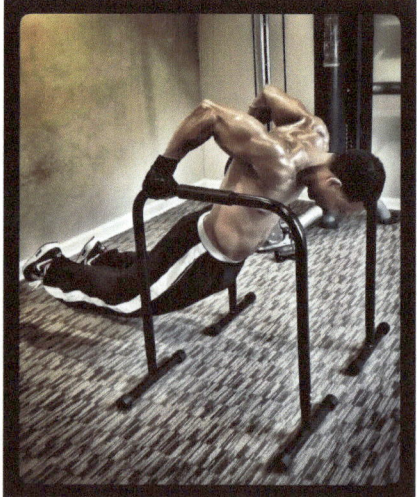

Variation #4
Wide Leg Dips
Muscles Worked: Triceps, Chest, Shoulders, Abdominals

How to:

1. Elevate your body up on the parallel bars with your arms fully extended, body tilted forward and your legs extended down spread widely. This is your starting positon.

2. Engage your core and slowly lower your body down by keeping your body titled forward and your legs continue to be spread widely. Breathe in and pause for a second at the bottom.

3. While breathing out, raise your body back up to the starting position.

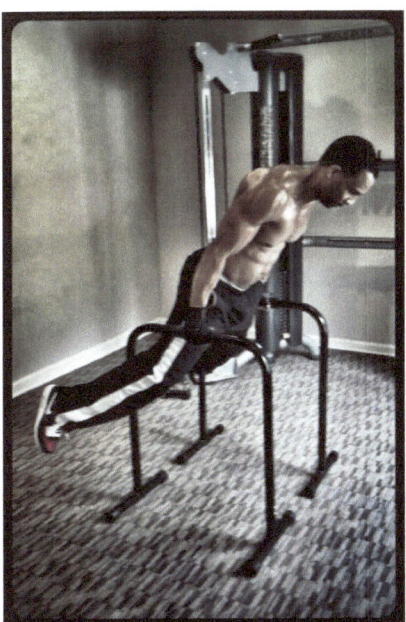
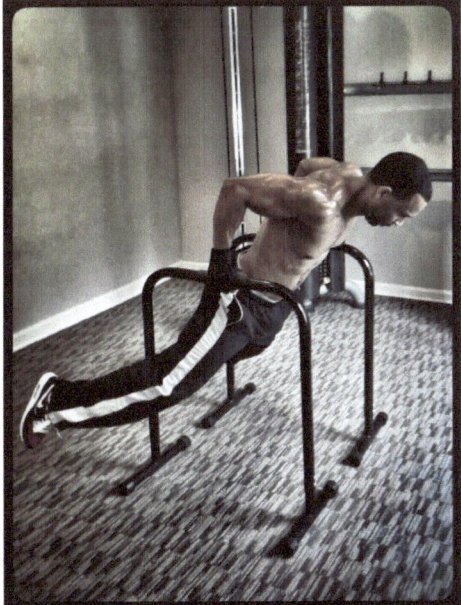

Variation #5
Cross Leg Style Dips
Muscles Worked: Triceps, Chest, Shoulders, Quads, Hamstrings

How to:

1. Elevate your body up over the parallel bars with your arms fully extended and your feet crossed in midair. This is your starting positon.

2. Engage your core and while breathing in slowly lower your body down while keeping your feet crossed in the starting position. Pause for a second at the bottom.

3. While breathing out, slowly raise your body back up to the starting position.

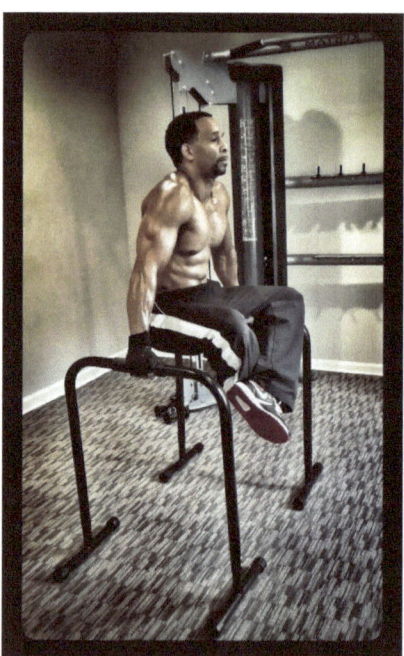 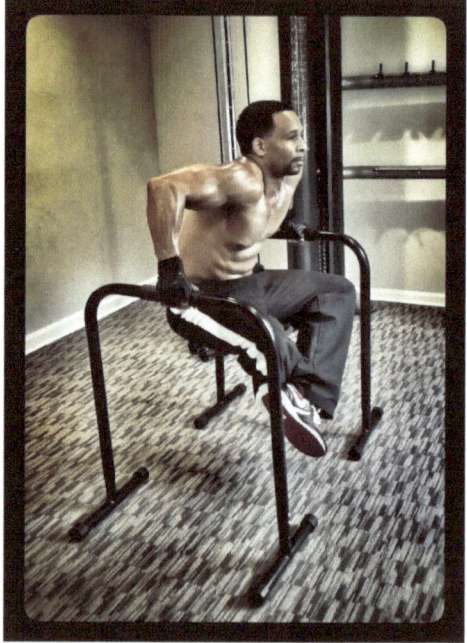

Variation #6
Tuck Leg Dips
Muscles Worked: Triceps, Chest, Shoulders, Quads, and Hamstrings

How to:
1. Elevate your body up over the parallel bars with your arms fully extended and your knees tucked into a 90 degree angle in midair. This is your starting positon.

2. Engage your core and while breathing in, slowly lower your body down while keeping your body in the tucked position. Pause for a second at the bottom.

3. While breathing out, slowly raise your body back up to the starting positon.

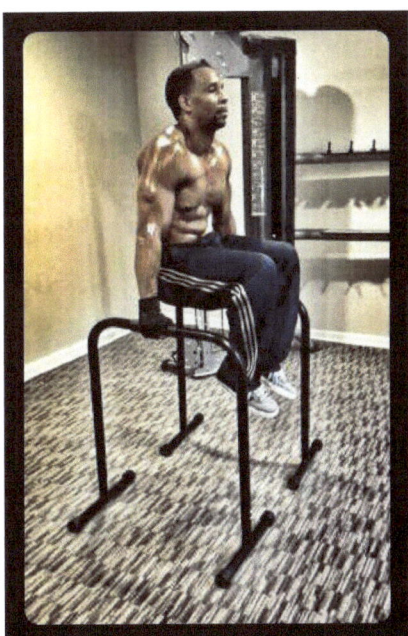 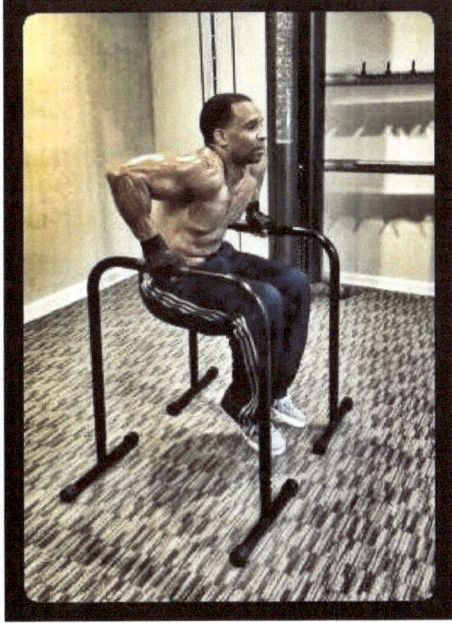

Variation #7
L-Sit Dips
Muscles Worked: Triceps, Chest, Abdominals, Quads, Hamstrings

How to:
1. Elevate your body up over the parallel bars with your arms fully extended and your legs extended outward until your body is in the L-Sit position or 90 degree angle in midair. This is your starting positon.

2. Engage your core and while breathing in, slowly lower your body back down while keeping your legs extended out in the L-Sit position in midair. Pause for a second at the bottom.

3. While breathing out, slowly raise your body back up to the starting position.

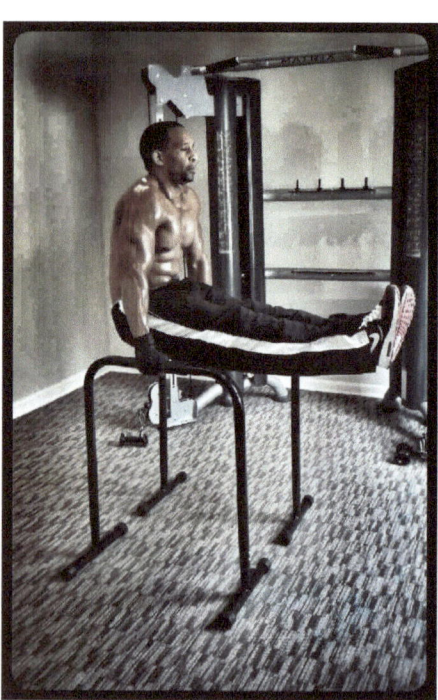 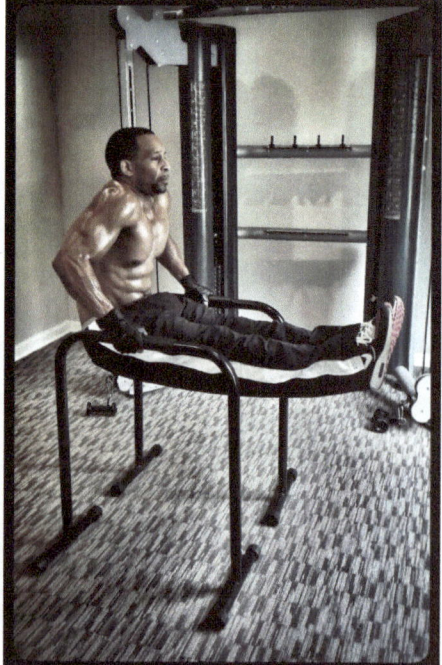

Variation #8
Bicycle Dips
Muscles Worked: Triceps, Chest, Abdominals, Quads, Hip Flexors

How to:
1. Elevate your body up over the parallel bars with your arms fully extended and your legs in the "bicycle pedaling" position in midair. This is your starting position.

2. Engage your core and while breathing in and out, slowly lower your body down then up while "bicycle pedaling" during each dip.

3. Your finish point is back to the starting position.

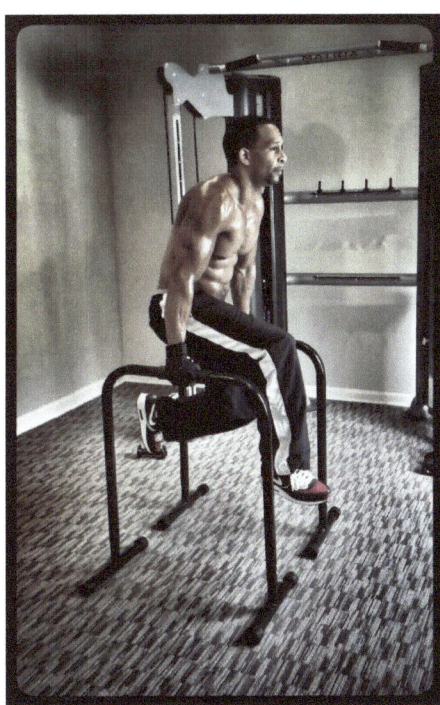 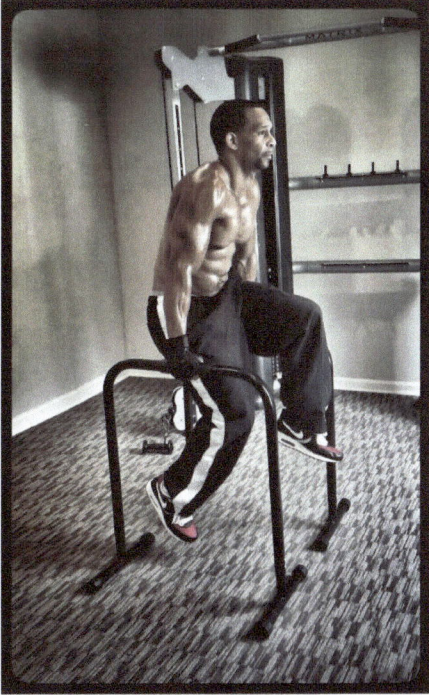

Variation #9
Dips to the Straddle Leg Raise
Muscles Worked: Triceps, Chest, Abdominals, Quads, Hamstrings

How to:

1. Position your body in the lower dip position with your knees bent and your feet together behind you without them being crossed. This is your starting position.

2. Engage your core and while breathing in, elevate your body up on top of the parallel bars with your arms fully extended and your legs straddled wide up over the bars.

3. While breathing out, lower your body back down slowly to the starting position.

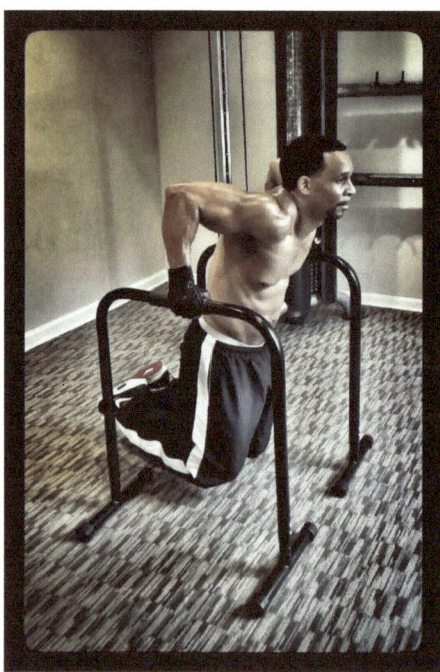 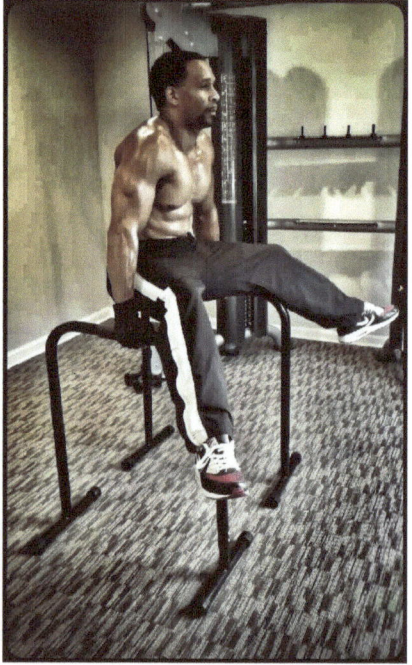

Chapter 2
L-Sit/V-Sit & Scissor/Bicycle Kicks:
Defined Six Pack, Ab Shredder and Strong Legs

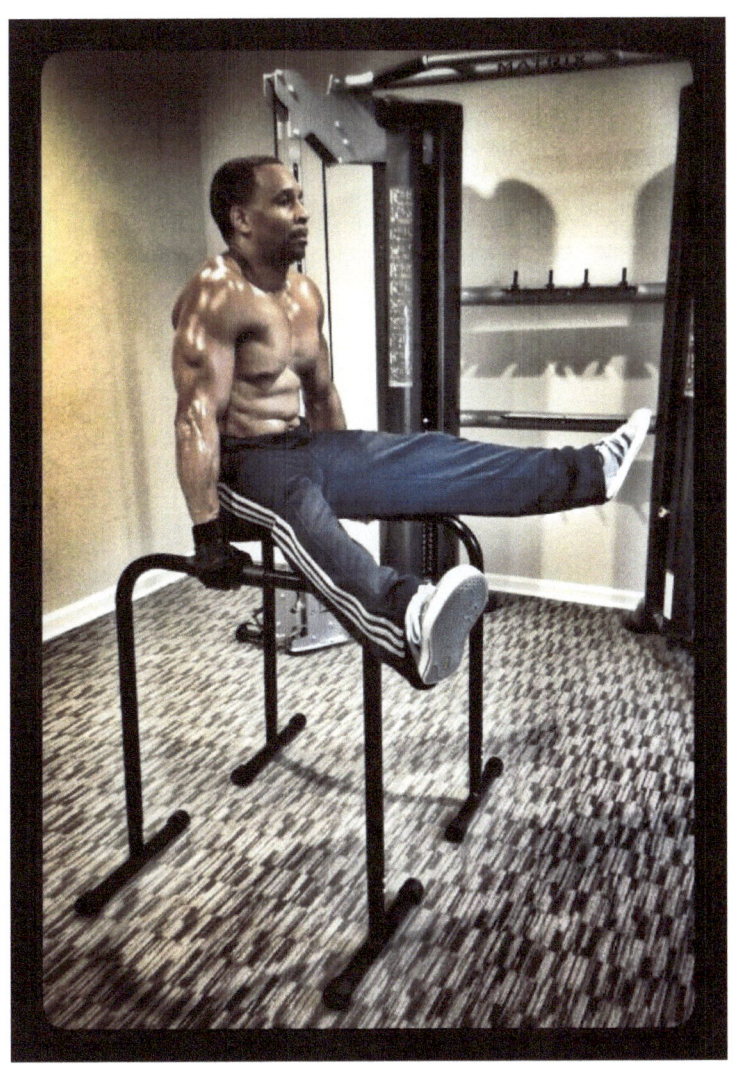

Variation #10
Leg Raise/L-Sit
Muscles Worked: Triceps, Abdominals, & Legs

How to:

1. Elevate your body up on top of the parallel bars with your arms fully extended and your legs fully extended down but your feet 1-2 inches off the floor. This is your starting position.

2. Engage your core and while breathing in, slowly raise your legs up to a 90 degree angle or the L-Sit position. Pause for a second at the L-Sit position.

3. While breathing out, slowly lower your legs back down to the starting position.

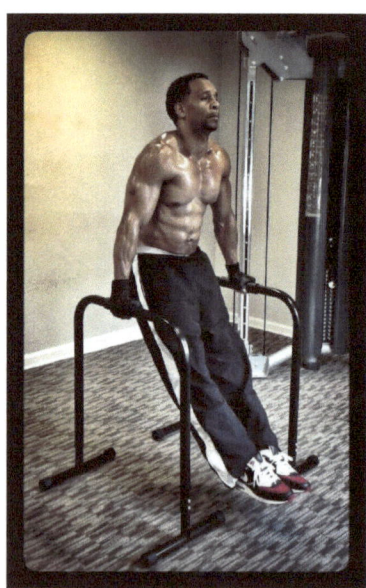 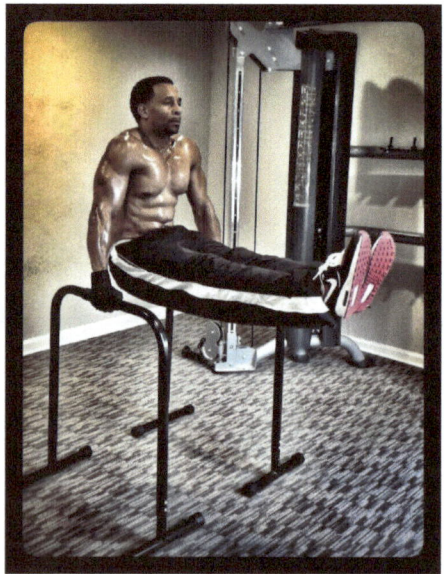

Variation #11
Side-to-Side L-Sit Swings
Muscles Worked: Triceps, Abdominals, Obliques, Legs

How to:
1. Elevate your body up on top of the parallel bars with your arms fully extended and your legs fully extended out in the L-Sit positon or 90-degree angle. This is your starting position.

2. Engage your core and while breathing in and out, slowly swing your legs from left to right by maintaining the L-Sit position. Pause for a second on each side swing.

3. After 15-25 swings, bring your legs to the middle of the bars and lower yourself down off the bars.

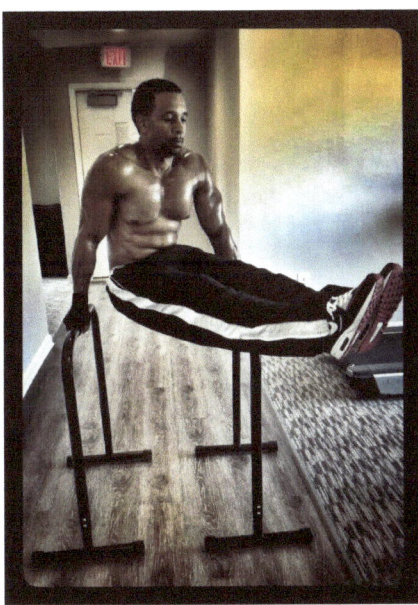 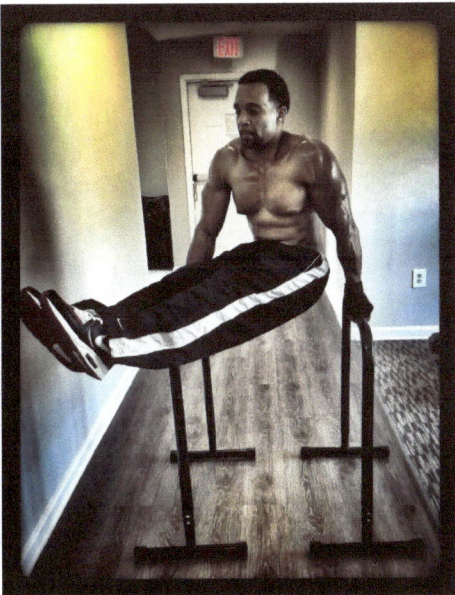

Variation #12
Tuck Planche to the V-Sit
Muscles Worked: Triceps, Abdominals, Shoulders, Legs

How to:
1. Elevate your body up on top of the parallel bars in a tuck position with your knees bent back so your feet are facing opposite your head. This is your starting position.

2. Engage your core and while breathing in, slowly swing your body forward in midair. Then once your legs start to reach the opposite direction, extend your legs out and up until you've reached the V-Sit position. Pause for a second at the top.

3. While breathing out, slowly retreat your body back to the tuck starting position.

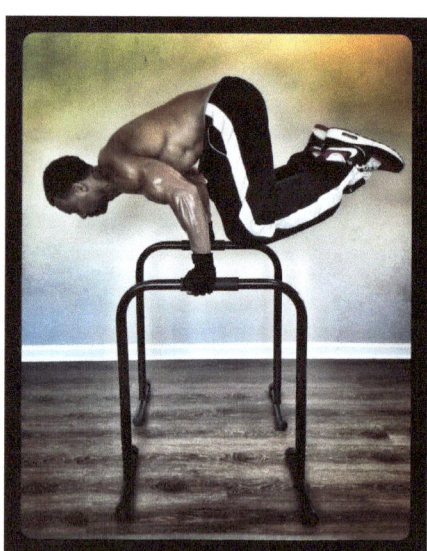 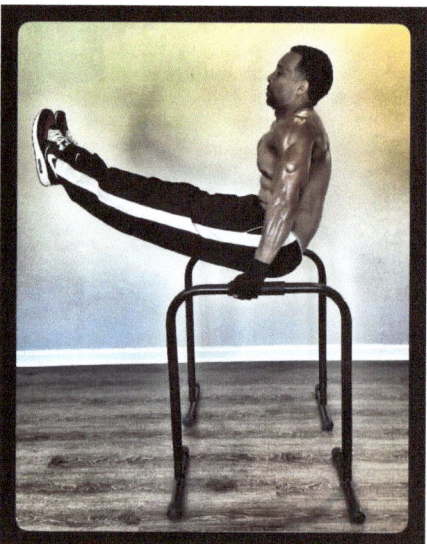

Variation #13
Wrist L-Sit
Muscles Worked: Forearms, Triceps, Shoulders, Abdominals, & Legs

How to:

1. Grab the ends of the parallel bars and place your forearms on top of the round edges of the bars. Prop your legs up then fully extend them straight out and together in the L-Sit position or 90-degree angle. This is your starting position.

2. Engage your core and while breathing in and out, hold the position for 20-30 seconds, depending on your fitness level.

3. Once finished, slowly lower your body off the bars.

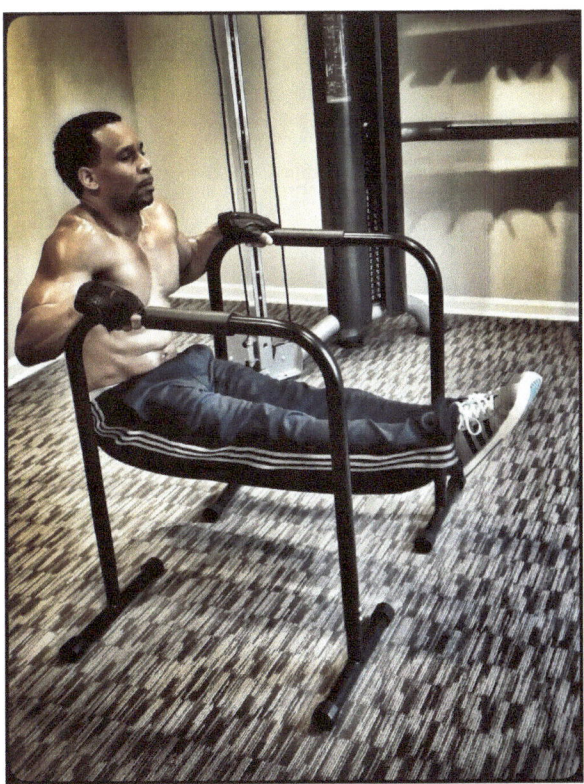

Variation #14
Wrist L-Sit Scissor Kicks
Muscles Worked: Forearms, Triceps, Shoulders, Abdominals, & Legs

How to:

1. Grab the ends of the parallel bars and place your forearms on top of the round edges of the bars. Prop your legs up the fully extend them straight out and together in the L-Sit position or 90-degree angle. This is your starting position.

2. Engage your core and while breathing in and out, start scissor kicking your legs while maintaining the L-Sit or 90-degree angle.

3. After 15-25 scissor kicks, depending on your fitness level, slowly bring both legs together to the starting position then lower your body off the bars.

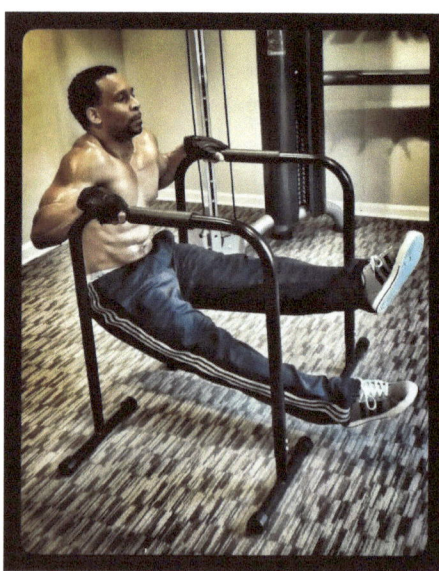 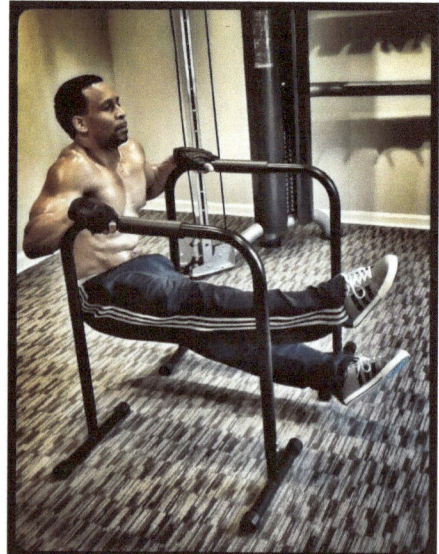

Variation #15
Top Bar Scissor Kicks
Muscles Worked: Triceps, Abdominals, & Legs

How to:

1. Elevate your body up on top of the parallel bars with your arms fully extended and your legs fully extended together out in the L-Sit position. This is your starting position.

2. Engage your core and while breathing in and out, start scissor kicking your legs while maintaining the L-Sit position or 90-degree angle.

3. After 15-25 scissor kicks, depending on the fitness level, slowly bring both legs together to the starting position then lower your body off the bars.

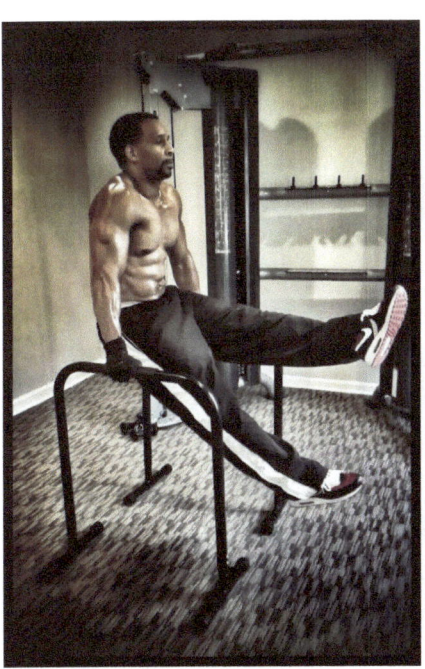
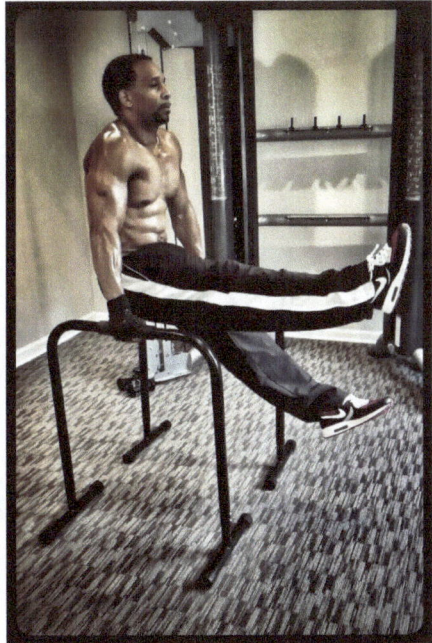

Variation #16
Low Horizontal In & Out L-Sit
Muscles Worked: Biceps, Abdominals, Quads, Hip Flexors, Hamstrings

How to:
1. Place your body on the inside of the parallel bars with your hands holding onto each bar with an underhand bicep grip. Pull your body all the way up into your biceps are locked and fully extend your legs out and together in the L-Sit position or the 90-degree angle. This is your starting position.

2. Engage your core and while breathing in and out, spread your legs in and out in the L-Sit position. Each in and out rep or swing, pause for one second.

3. Once finished, slowly lower your body off the bars.

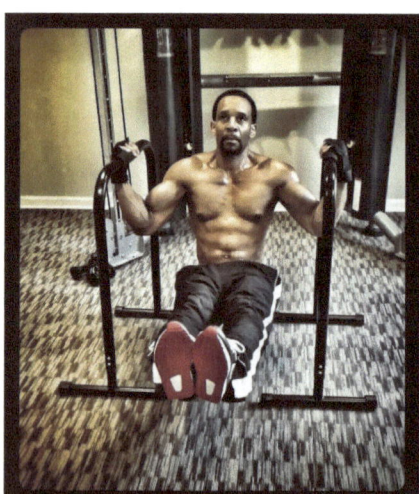 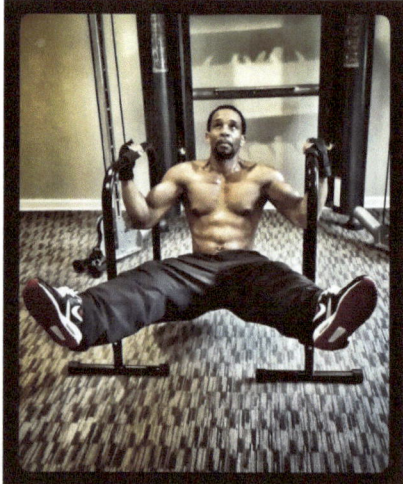

Variation #17
Elbow L-Sit
Muscles Worked: Forearms, Triceps, Abdominals, & Legs

How to:

1. Prop your body up on top of the parallel bars by resting your forearms and elbows on top of the bar while fully extending your legs out and together in the L-Sit position or 90-degree angle. This is your starting position.

2. Engage your core and while breathing in and out, maintain that same position for 20-30 seconds depending on your fitness level.

3. When finished, slowly lower your body off the bars.

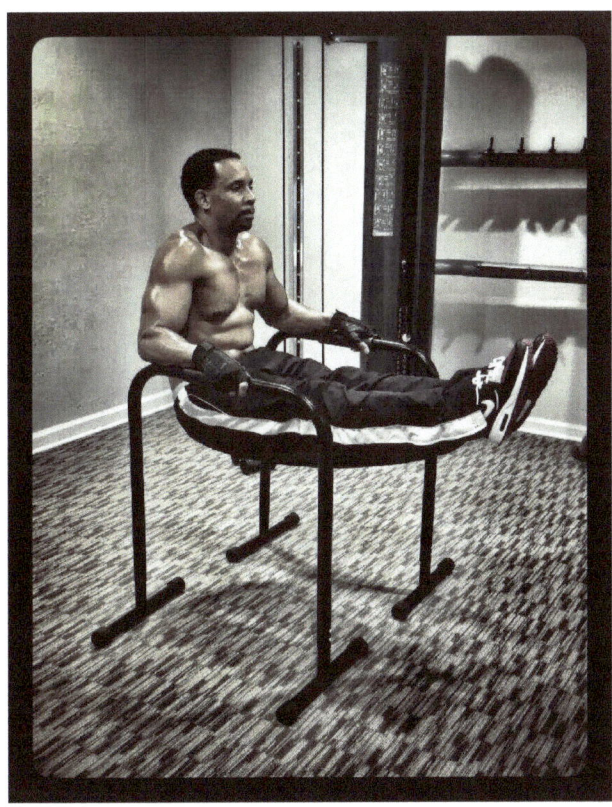

Variation #18
Horizontal Front Lever Scissor Kicks
Muscles Worked: Biceps, Abdominals, Hip Flexors & Legs

How to:
1. Lay your body on the inside of the parallel bars with your hands holding onto each bar with an underhand bicep grip. Pull your body up in the front lever position with your left leg fully extended all the way up and your right leg fully extended out. This is your starting position.

2. Engage your core and while breathing in and out, start the scissor kick motion with your legs while maintaining the front lever position with your body.

3. After 15-25 scissor kicks, depending on your fitness level, slowly lower your body back down off the bars.

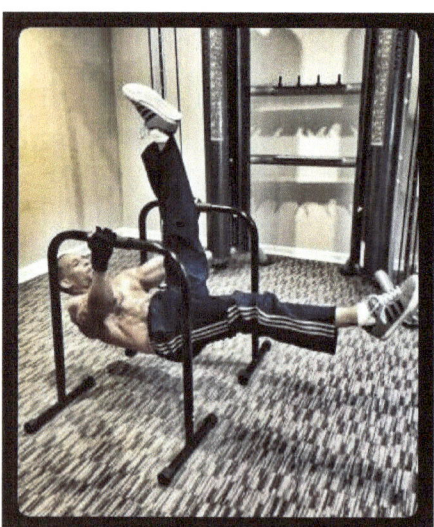 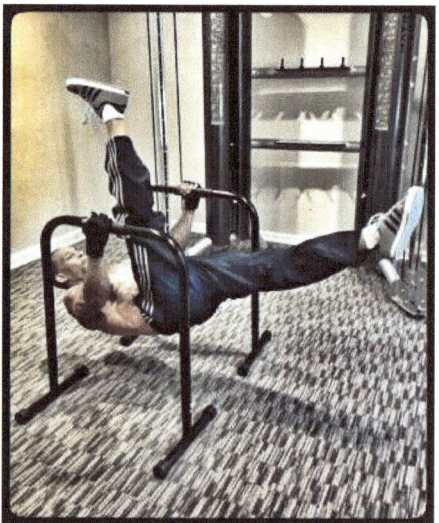

Variation #19
Top Bar In & Out L-Sit
Muscles Worked: Triceps, Abdominals, Quads, Hamstrings, Hip Flexors

How to:
1. Elevate your body up over the parallel bars with your arms fully extended and your legs extended outwards until your body is in the L-Sit position or 90-degree angle in midair. This is your starting position.

2. Engage your core and while breathing in and out, open and close your legs in and out while maintaining your body in the L-Sit position or 90-degree angle. Each in and out rep, pause for one second.

3. After 15-25 in and out reps, depending on your fitness level, lower your body back down off the bars.

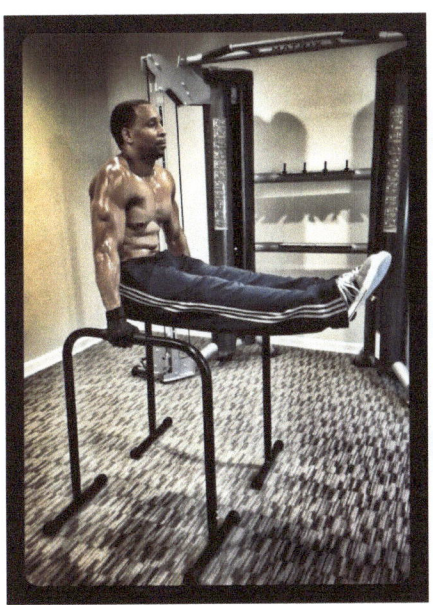 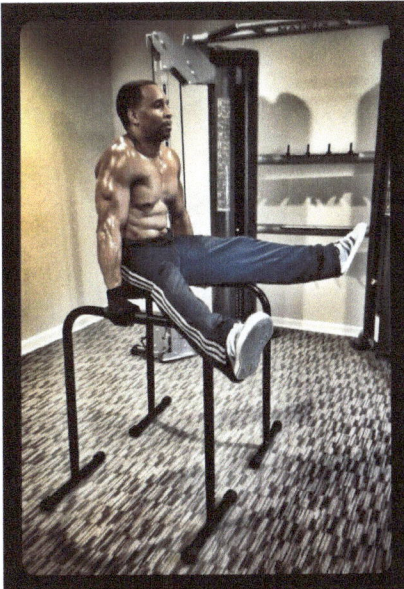

Variation #20
Horizontal Front Lever Bicycle Kicks
Muscles Worked: Biceps, Abdominals, Hip Flexors & Legs

How to:

1. Lay your body on the inside of the parallel bars with your hands holding onto each bar with an underhand bicep grip. Pull your body up in the front lever position with your left leg tucked towards your chest and your right leg fully extended out. This is your starting position.

2. Engage your core and while breathing in and out, start the bicycle kicking motion with your legs while maintaining the front lever position with your body.

3. After 15-25 bicycle kicks, depending on your fitness level, slowly lower your body back down off the bars.

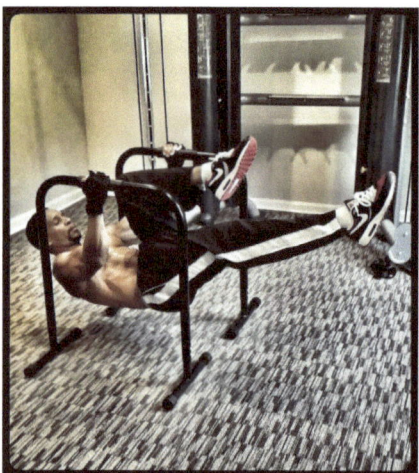 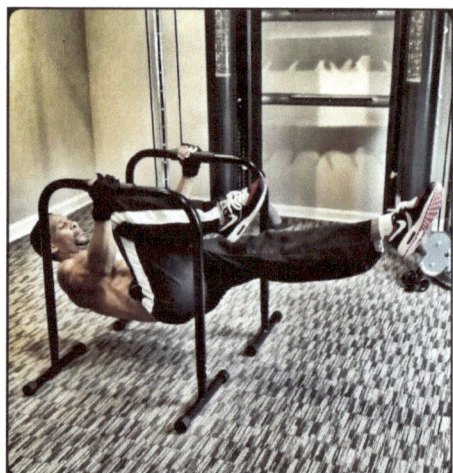

Chapter 3
Pull Ups/Chin Ups/Muscle Ups:
Broad and Defined Shoulders and Back

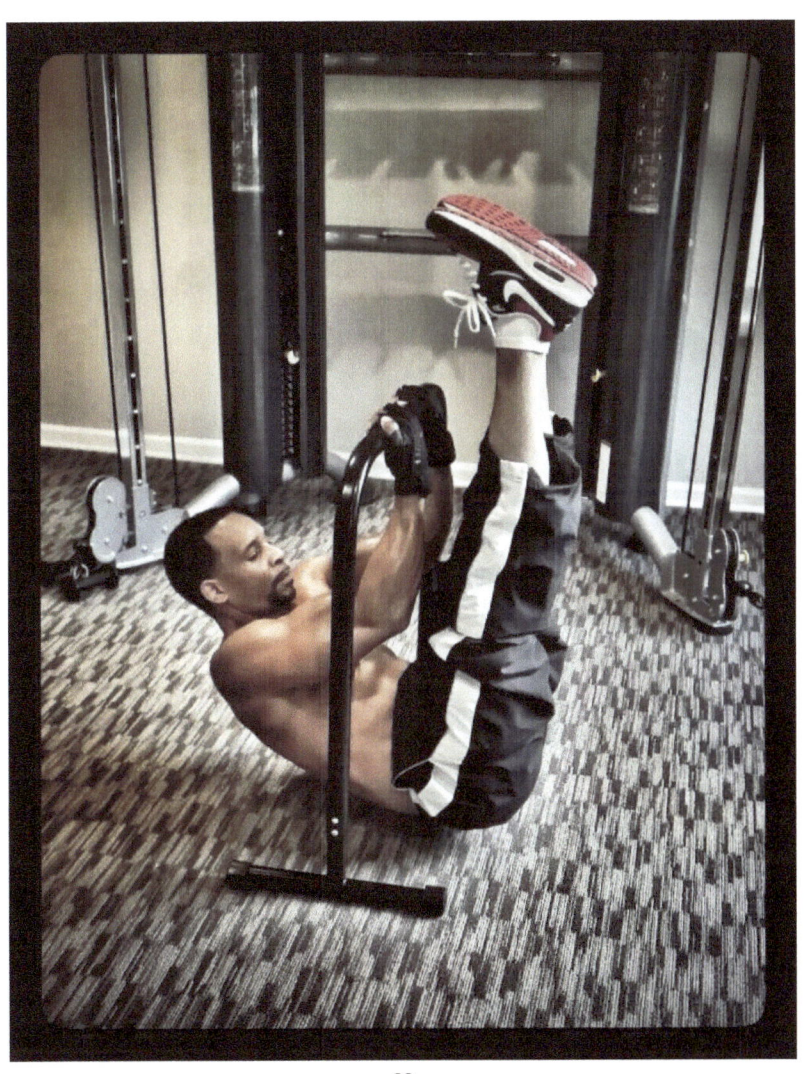

Variation #21
Horizontal Pull-Ups
Muscles Worked: Biceps, Back, Abdominals

How to:

1. Lay your body on the inside of the parallel bars with your hands holding onto each bar with an underhand bicep grip. Your legs should be fully extended out with only your heels touching the floor. This is your starting position.

2. Engage your core and while breathing in, pull your body all the way up until your biceps are locked. Squeeze your back and bicep and pause for one second at the top.

3. While breathing out, slowly lower your body back down to the starting position.

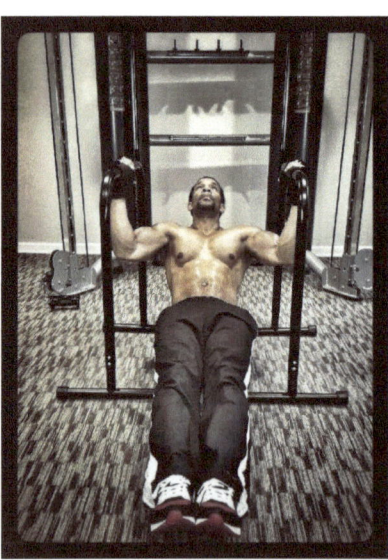 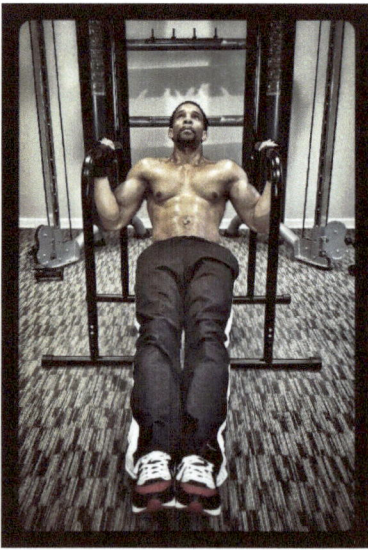

Variation #22
V-Up Horizontal Pull Ups
Muscles Worked: Biceps, Back, Abdominals, & Legs

How to:
1. Lay your body on the inside of the parallel bars with your hands holding onto each bar with an underhand bicep grip. Pull your body up off the floor about one inch and raise your fully extended legs to the V-Up position. This is your starting position.

2. Engage your core and while breathing in, pull your body all the way up until your biceps are locked and your body maintained in the V-Up position. Squeeze your back and bicep and pause for one second at the top.

3. While breathing out, slowly lower your body back down to the starting position.

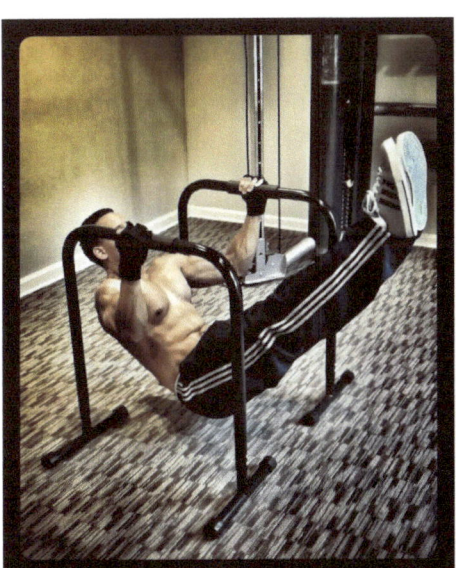 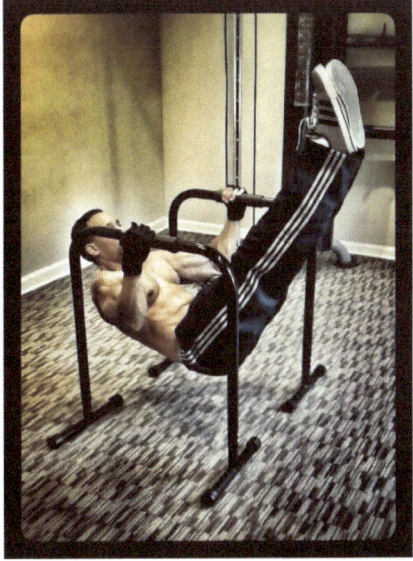

Variation #23
Horizontal Low L-Sit to the L-Up Pull Up
Muscles Worked: Biceps, Back, Abdominals, & Legs

How to:
1. Lay your body on the inside of the parallel bars with your hands holding onto each bar with an underhand bicep grip. Pull your body up off the floor about one inch and fully extend your legs together out in the L-Sit position. This is your starting position.

2. Engage your core and while breathing in, pull your body all the way up until your biceps are locked and your body forms a backward "L" shape. Squeeze your back and biceps and pause for one second at the top.

3. While breathing out, slowly lower your body back down to the starting position.

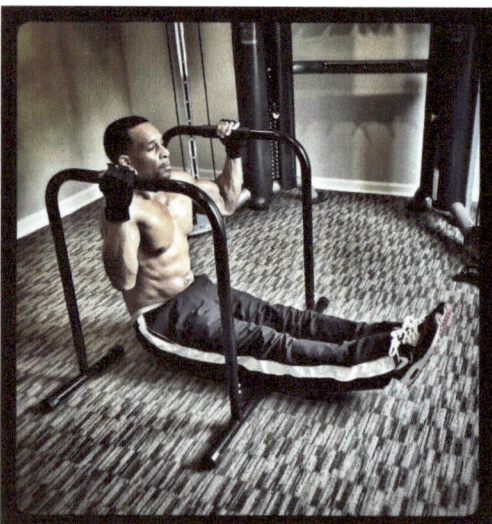 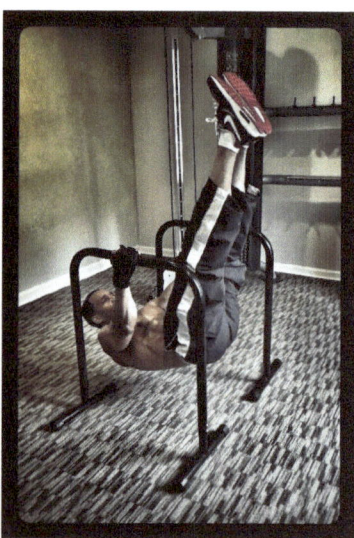

Variation #24
Single Bar L-Sit Chin Ups
Muscles Worked: Biceps, Back, Abdominals, & Legs

How to:

1. Place your body through the single parallel bar and grab the top of the bar with an underhand bicep grip. Pull your body up off the floor about one inch and fully extend your legs together out in the L-Sit position. This is your starting position.

2. Engage your core and while breathing in, pull your body up until your chin is completely over the bar. Continue to keep your legs in the L-Sit position throughout the movement. Pause for one second at the top.

3. While breathing out, slowly lower your body back down to the starting position.

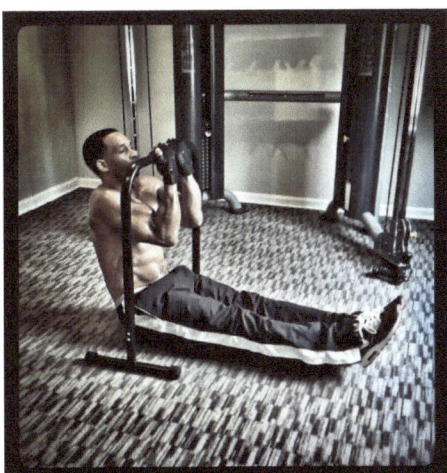 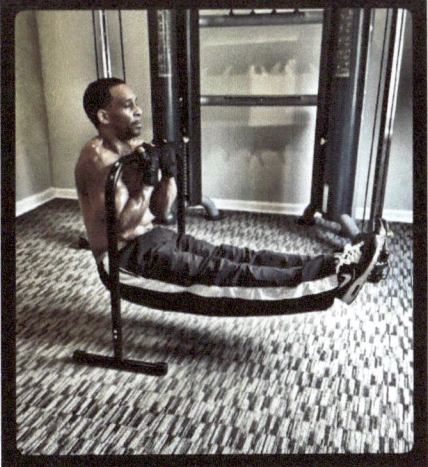

Variation #25
Single Bar Bicep L-Ups
Muscles Worked: Forearms, Biceps, Back, Abdominals, & Legs

How to:
1. Place your body through the single parallel bar and grab the top of the bar with an underhand bicep grip. Pull your body up off the floor about one inch and lift your legs all the way up until your body is in the backwards L-Sit position. This is your starting position.

2. Engage your core and while breathing in, pull your body all the way up until it forms a backwards elevated L-Sit position. Keep your legs together and straight with your toes pointed out. Pause for one second at the top.

3. While breathing out, lower your body slowly back down to the starting position.

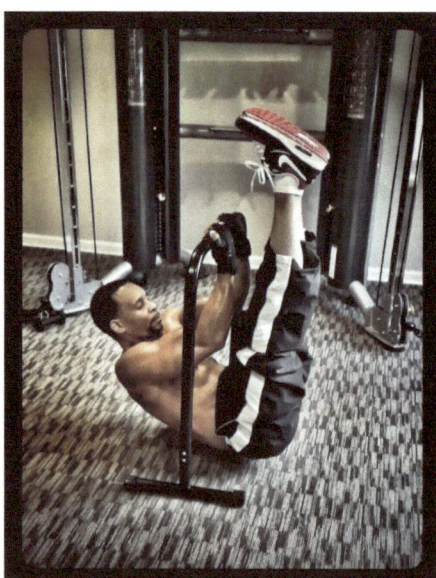 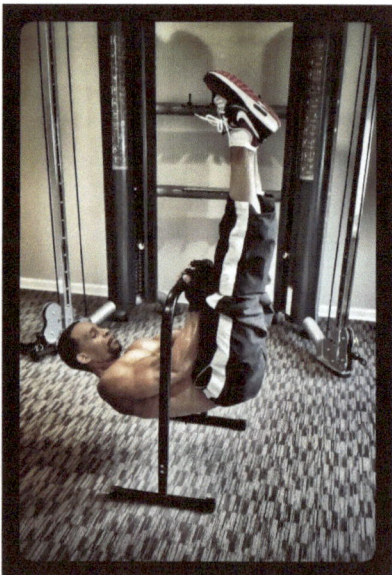

Variation #26
Elbow L-Sit to the Elbow V-Up
Muscles Worked: Forearms, Triceps, Abdominals, & Legs

How to:

1. Prop your body up on top of the parallel bars by resting your forearms and elbows on top of the bars while fully extending your legs out and together in the L-Sit position or 90-degree angle. This is your starting position.

2. Engage your core and while breathing in, elevate your legs up to the V-Up position. Hold that position for one second.

3. While breathing out, slowly lower your legs back down to the starting position.

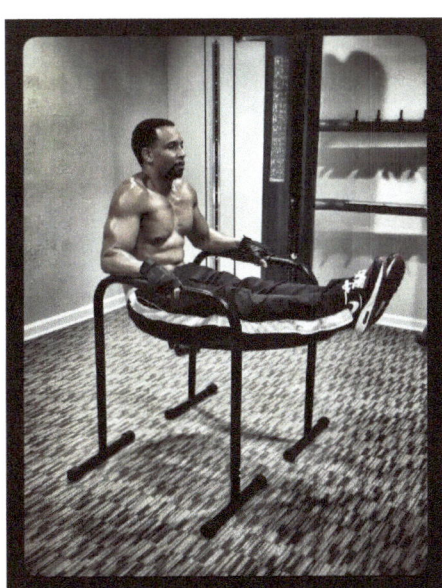 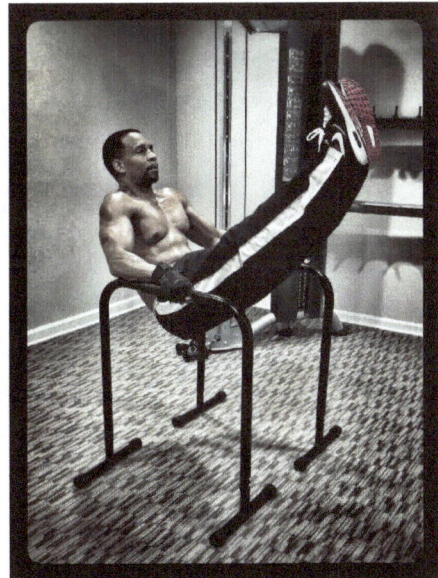

Variation #27
Single Bar Muscle Ups
Muscles Worked: Forearms, Biceps, Triceps, Chest, Back, & Abdominals

How to:

1. Position your body in between a single bar. Grab the bar with an overhand grip. Raise your body up until your chin clears the top of the bar and your legs extended out with a slight bend at the knee area. This is your starting position.

2. Engage your core and while breathing in, slowly and carefully muscle your body up over the bar with your arms fully extended and your feet about 1-2 inches off the floor. *Note: Do not jerk your body during the muscle up movement because you must keep the single bar balanced and stabilized at all times.*

3. While breathing out, slowly lower your body back down to the starting position.

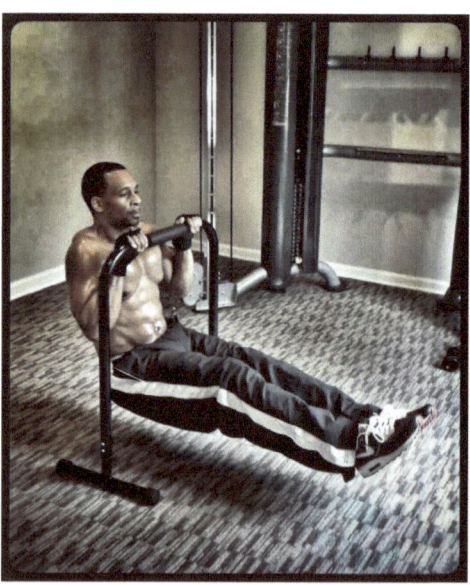 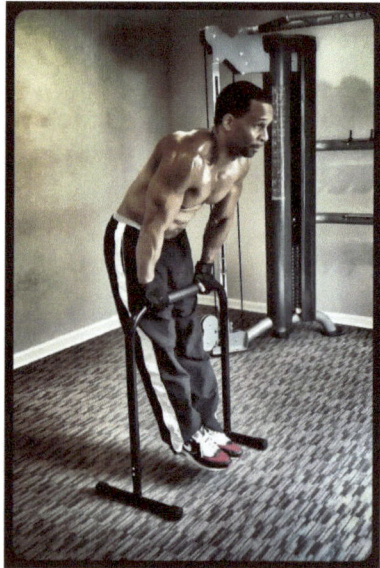

Chapter 4
Push Ups: Ultimate Chest Blaster

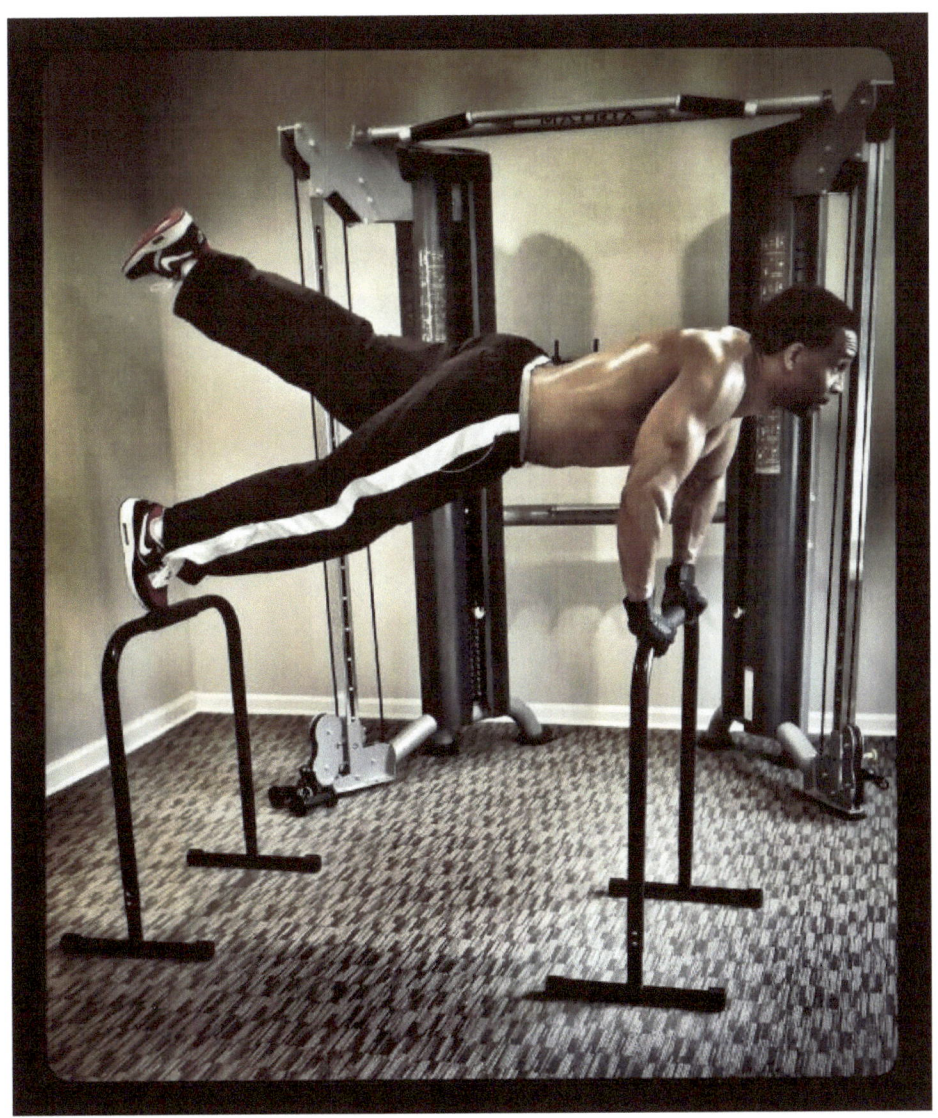

Variation #28
Tuck Planche Push Up
Muscles Worked: Triceps, Chest, Shoulders, Abdominals

How to:
1. Raise your body into the tuck position on the parallel bars with your knees bent and feet behind you. Make sure your torso and head are positioned parallel to the bars. This is your starting position.

2. Engage your core and while breathing in, push your tucked positioned body up with your arms fully extended. Pause at the top for one second.

3. While breathing out, lower your body back down to the starting position.

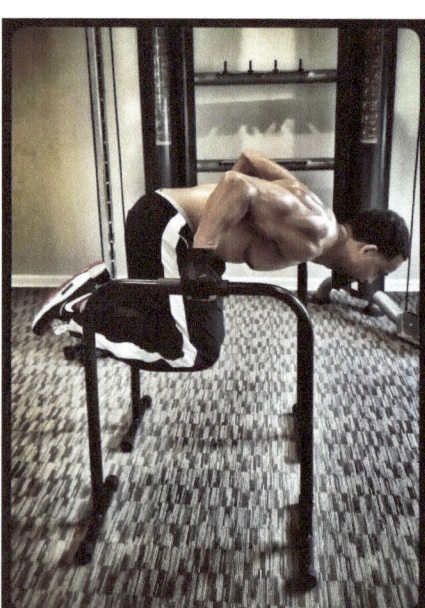
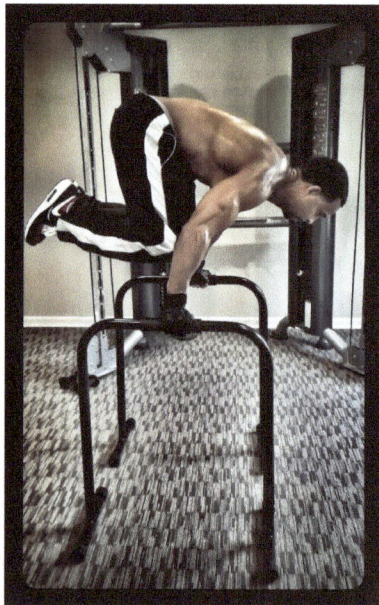

Variation #29
Standing/Leaning Parallel Bar Push Ups
Muscles Worked: Chest, Triceps, Abdominals, Shoulders

How to:
1. In a standing/leaning forward position, grab the top rounded edges of the parallel bars with your arms fully extended while standing on your toes. This is your starting position.

2. Engage your core and while breathing in, lower your body forward and down in the deep push up position with your torso in between the parallel bars. Pause for one second at the bottom.

3. While breathing out, slowly raise your body back up to the starting position.

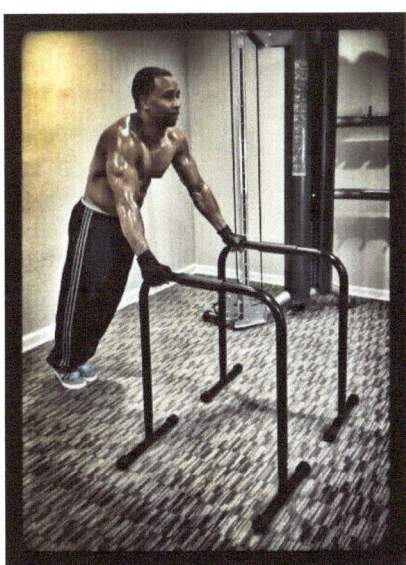 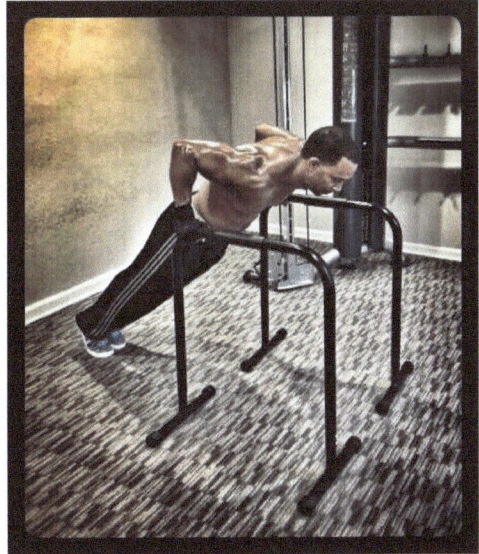

Variation #30
Top Bar Push Ups
Muscles Worked: Chest, Triceps, Abdominals, Shoulders

How to:

1. Elevate your body on top of both bars in the push up position with your arms fully extended up. This is your starting position.

2. Engage your core and while breathing in, lower your body down until your chest taps the bar. Pause for one second at the bottom. *Note: Maintain extreme focus with your stabilization muscles to keep your body and the bars balanced.*

3. While breathing out, raise your body back up to the starting position.

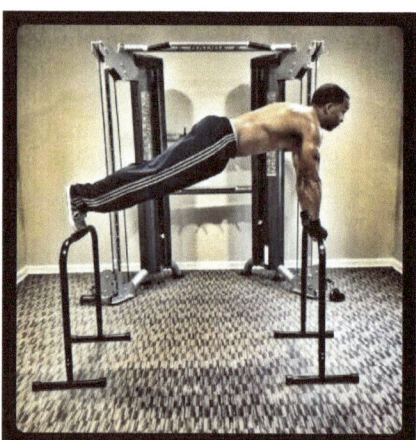 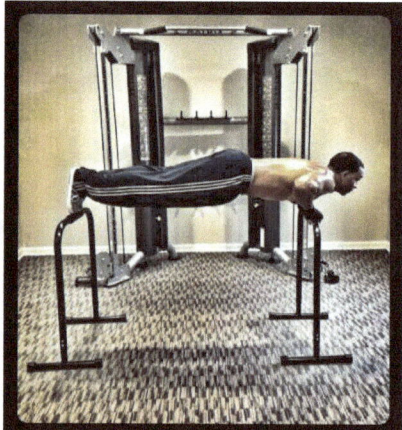

Variation #31
Elevated Leg Top Bar Push Ups
Muscles Worked: Chest, Triceps, Shoulders, Abdominals, & Hamstrings

How to:
1. Elevate your body on top of both bars in the push up position. Lift one leg up with your arms fully extended up. This is your starting position.

2. Engage your core and while breathing in lower your body down until your chest taps the bar. Keep your one leg elevated and pause for one second at the bottom. *Note: Maintain extreme focus with your stabilization muscles to keep your body and the bars balanced.*

3. While breathing out raise your body back up to the starting position.

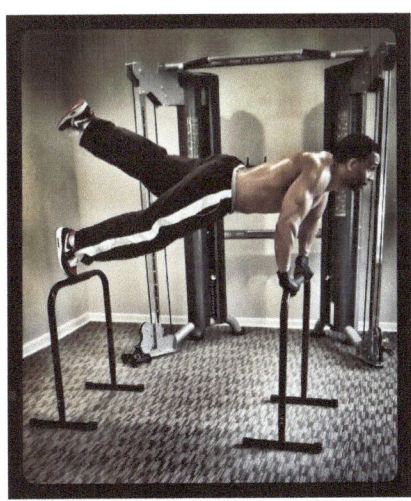 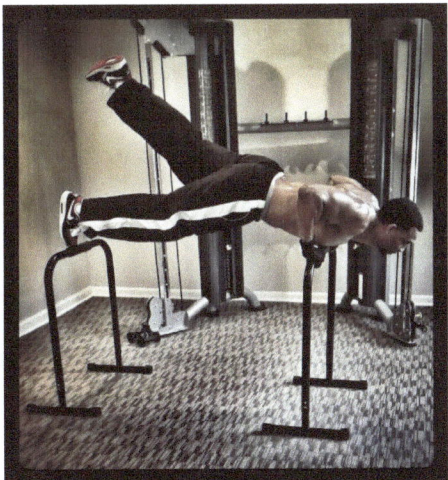

Variation #32
Hand Stand Push Up
Muscles Worked: Triceps, Shoulders, Back, Abdominals, & Legs

How to:
1. Place your body in the lower hand stand position by balancing your entire body with your shoulders, abdominals and legs in midair. This is your starting position. *Note: If you're not strong enough, you can perform this same exercise with your feet propped up against the wall.*

2. Engage your core and while breathing in push your body straight up in the air until your arms and legs are fully extended up. Pause for a second at the top.

3. While breathing out, slowly lower your body back down to the starting position.

<u>Wall Version</u>

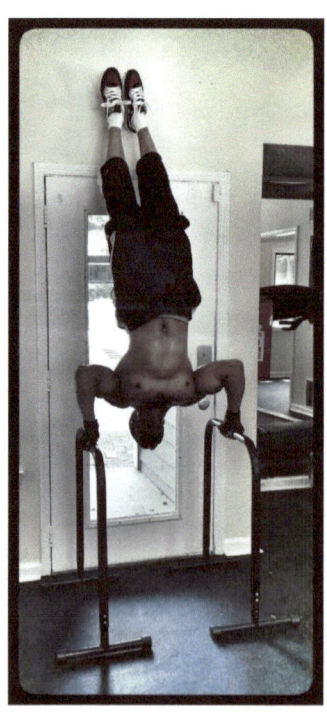
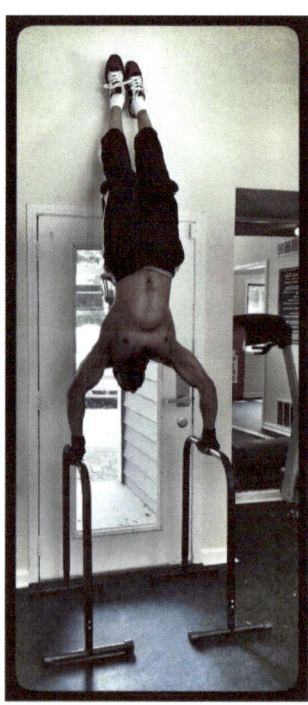

<u>Mid-Air Version</u>

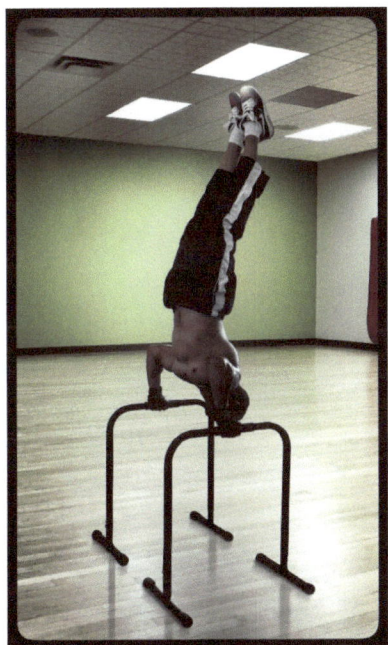 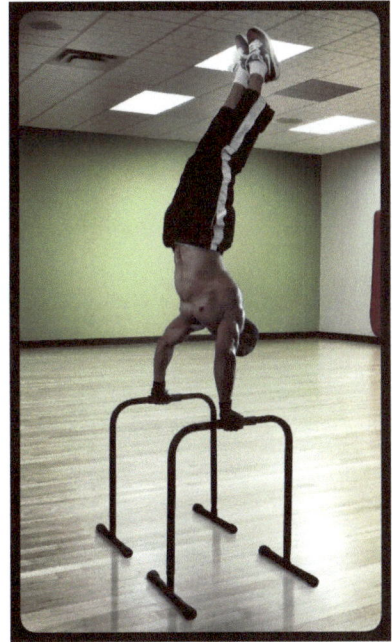

Note: *Use extreme caution when doing the mid-air handstand push up on the parallel bars. It takes extreme balance, stabilization, and core strength to complete this exercise properly.*

Chapter 5
Planche/Supermans: Best Total Body Physique

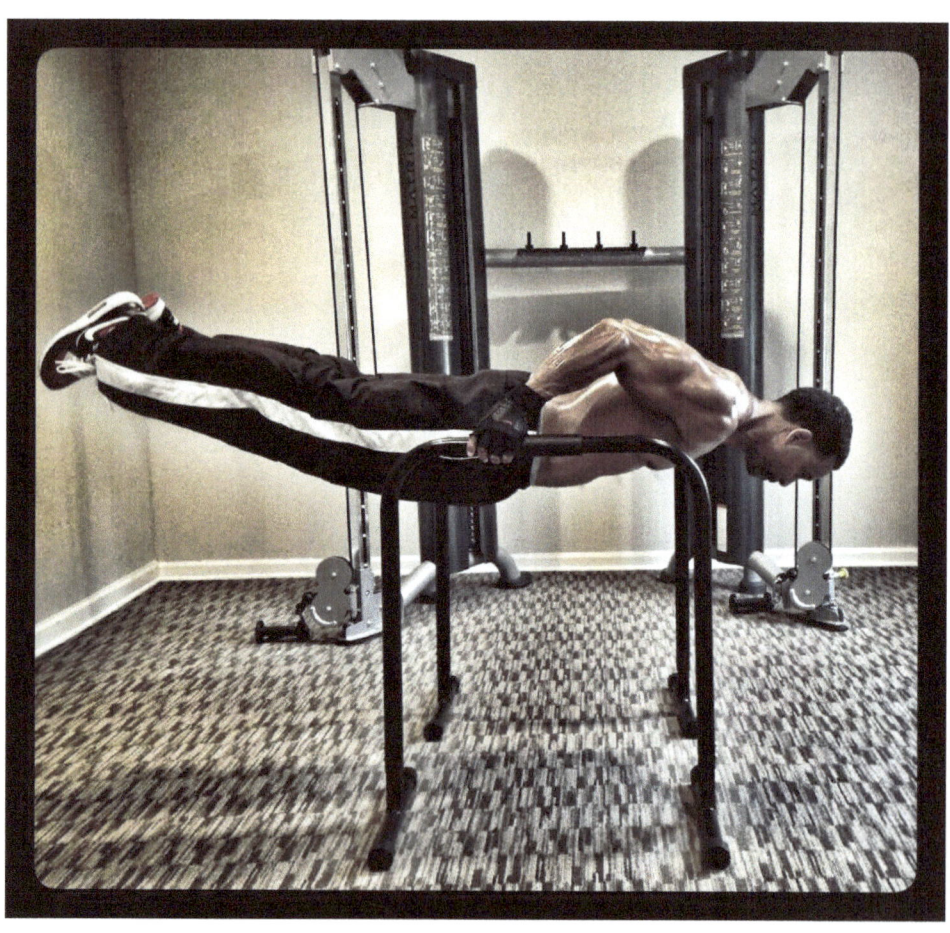

Variation #33
Extended Leg Elevated Planche Raise
Muscles Worked: Triceps, Abdominals, Shoulders, & Legs

How to:

1. Elevate your body up on top of the parallel bars with your arms fully extended and your legs fully extended down while your feet are 1-2 inches off the floor. Make sure your back is slightly rounded at the top. This is your starting position.

2. Engage your core and while breathing in, elevate your body up by using your abdominal muscles to position your body like the number "7" or the backwards number "7". Pause for one second at the top.

3. While breathing out, slowly lower your body back down to the starting position.

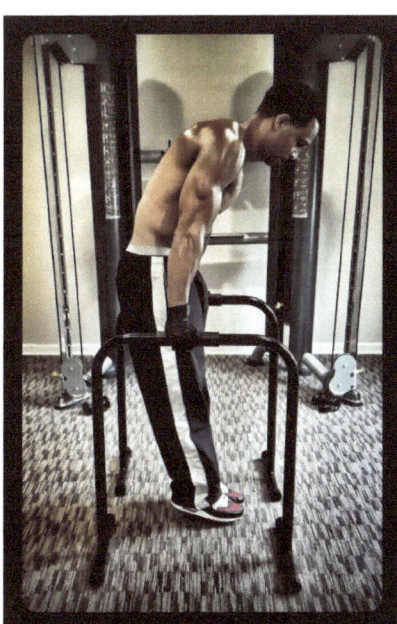 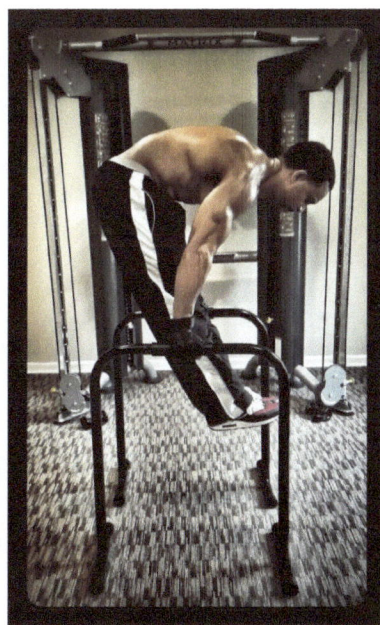

Variation #34
Top L-Sit to the Superman Wide Leg Dive
Muscles Worked: Triceps, Abdominals, Shoulders, & Legs

How to:

1. Elevate your body up over the parallel bars with your arms fully extended and your legs fully extended outward until your body is in the L-Sit position or 90-degree angle in midair. This is your starting position.

2. Engage your core and while breathing in, tuck your legs underneath your torso and continue to slowly swing them behind you with your legs spread wide apart. Your body should end up in a planche dive position. Hold this position for about 5-10 seconds.

3. While breathing out, reverse your body's movement back to the starting L-Sit position or 90-degree angle.

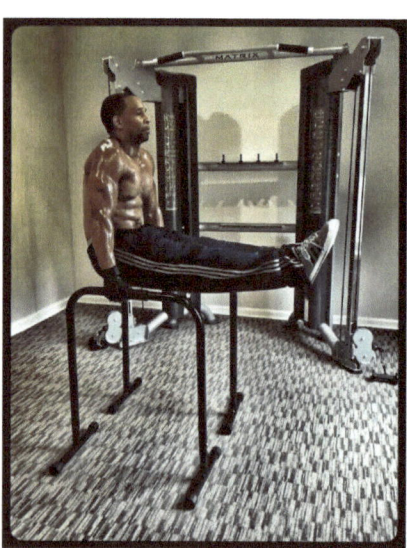 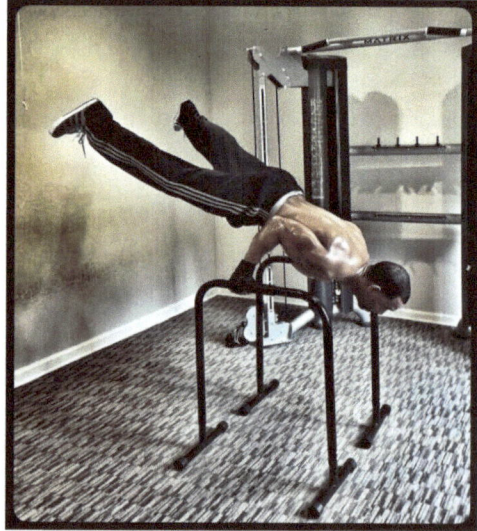

Variation #35
<u>L-Sit Raise to the Tuck Planche</u>
Muscles Worked: Triceps, Chest, Abdominals, Shoulders

How to:
1. Elevate your body up over the parallel bars with your arms fully extended and your legs fully extended outward until your body is in the L-Sit position or 90-degree angle in midair. This is your starting position.

2. Engage your core and while breathing in, tuck your legs underneath your torso until your body is completely in the tuck position with your knees bent and feet behind. Hold this position for about 5-10 seconds.

3. While breathing out, reverse your body's movement back to the starting L-Sit position or 90-degree angle.

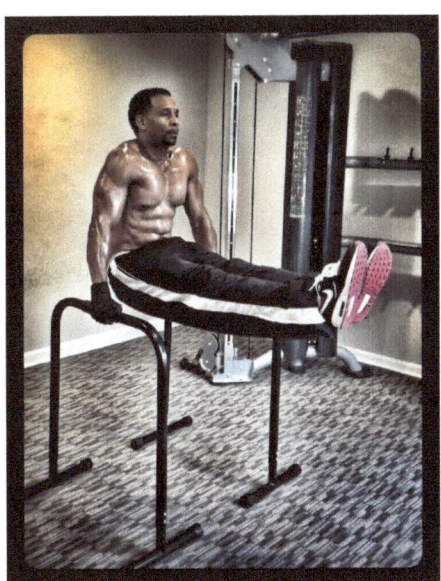 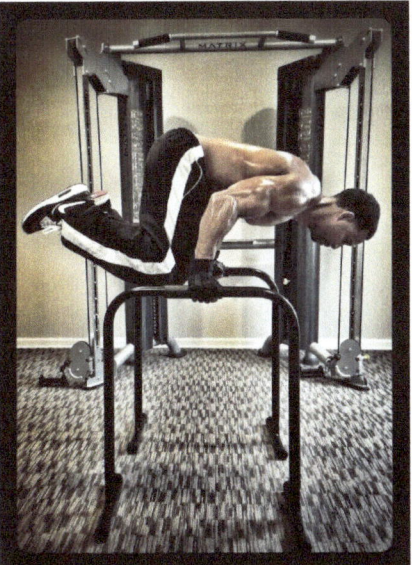

Variation #36
Top L-Sit to the Superman Stance
Muscles Worked: Triceps, Chest, Abdominals, Shoulders, & Legs

How to:

1. Elevate your body up over the parallel bars with your arms fully extended and your legs fully extended outward until your body is in the L-Sit position or 90-degree angle in midair. This is your starting position.

2. Engage your core and while breathing in, tuck your legs underneath your torso and continue to slowly swing them behind you until your body is in the full planche or superman position. Hold this position for about 5-10 seconds.

3. While breathing out, reverse your body's movement back to the starting L-Sit position or 90-degree angle.

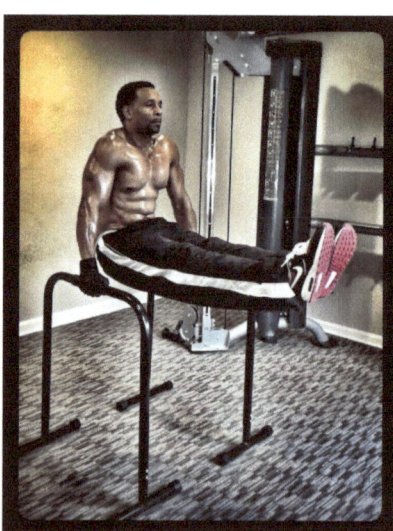 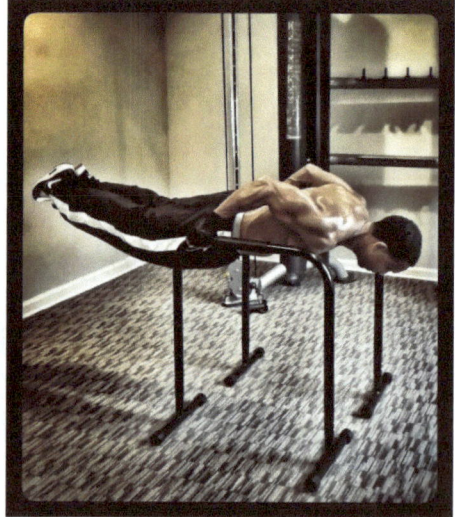

Variation #37
Tuck Planche to the Superman Position
Muscles Worked: Triceps, Chest, Abdominals, Shoulders, & Legs

How to:
1. Raise your body into the tuck position on the parallel bars with your knees bent behind you. Make sure your torso and head are aligned parallel to the bars. This is your starting position.

2. Engage your core and while breathing in, slowly swing your legs behind you until your body is in the full planche or superman position. Hold this position for about 5-10 seconds.

3. While breathing out, reverse your body's movement back to the tuck planche position.

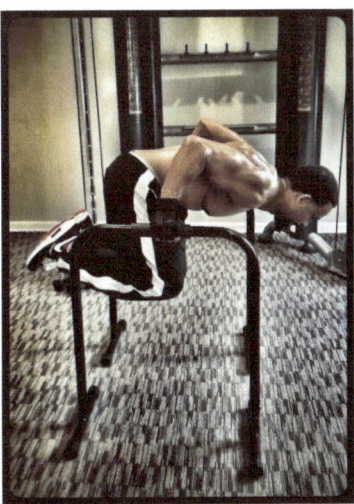 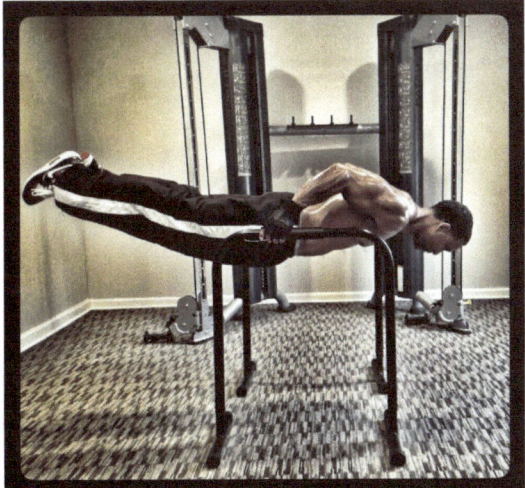

Variation #38
Single Bar Superman Stance
Muscles Worked: Triceps, Abdominals, Shoulders, & Legs

How to:

1. Lay a single parallel bar onto the floor with the top handle touching the floor. Place your grip near the end of the bar and lean your torso forward with your knees bent and feet on the floor.

2. Engage your core and while breathing in and out, slowly swing your legs up and back behind you until your body is in the full planche or superman position. Hold this position for about 5-10 seconds.

3. When finished lower your body off the bars.

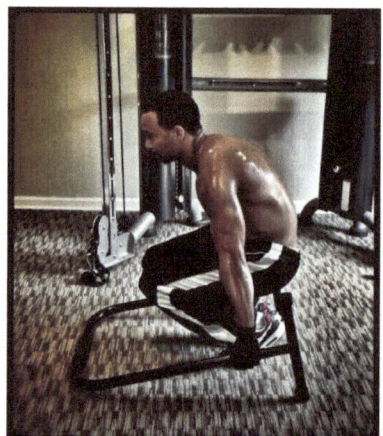

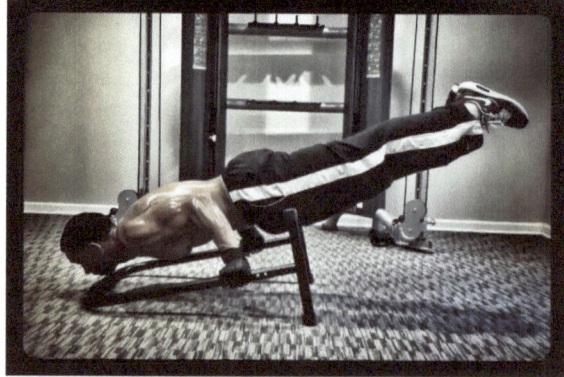

Variation #39
Tuck Planche to the Superman Dive
Muscles Worked: Triceps, Abdominals, Shoulders, & Legs

How to:

1. Raise your body into the tuck position on the parallel bars with your knees behind you. Make sure your torso and head are aligned parallel to the bars. This is your starting position.

2. Engage your core and while breathing in, slowly swing your legs behind you until they are fully in the superman dive position with your legs tilted up. Hold this position for about 5-10 seconds.

3. While breathing out, reverse your body's movement back to the tuck planche position.

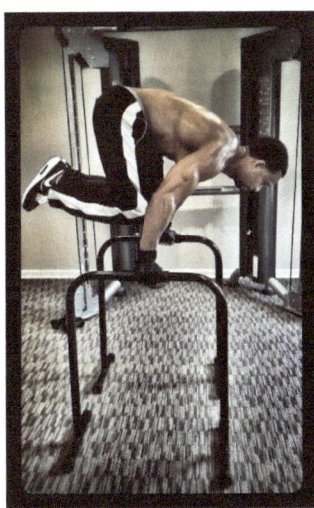 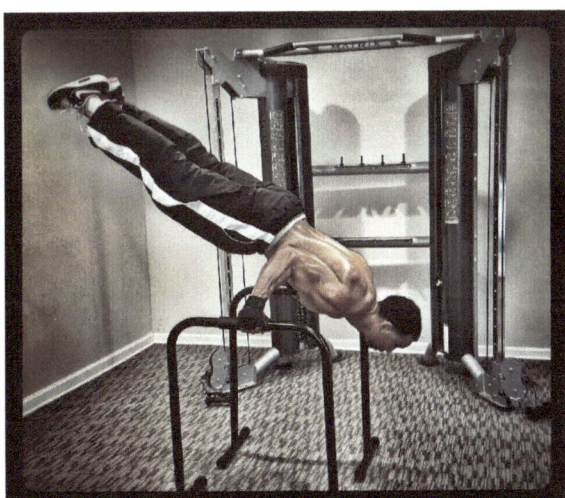

Variation #40
Wrist L-Sit to the Superman Wide Leg Dive
Muscles Worked: Forearms, Triceps, Abdominals, Shoulders, & Legs

How to:
1. Grab the ends of the parallel bars and place your forearms on top of the round edges of the bars. Prop your legs up then fully extend them straight out and together in the L-Sit position or 90-degree angle. This is your starting position.

2. Engage your core and while breathing in, muscle your forearm and wrist off the bar then slowly swing your leg behind you and in the tilt full-planche dive or superman dive. Spread your legs apart. Hold this position for about 5-10 seconds.

3. While breathing out, reverse your body's movement back to the wrist L-Sit starting position.

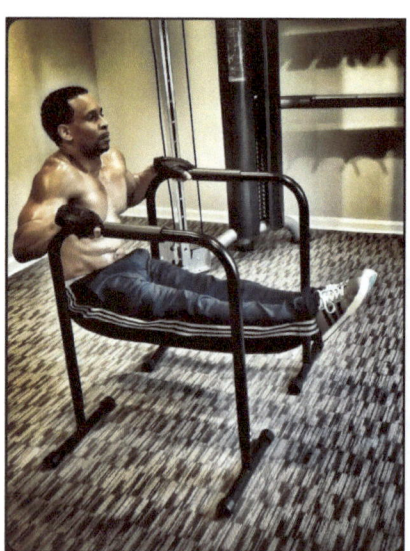 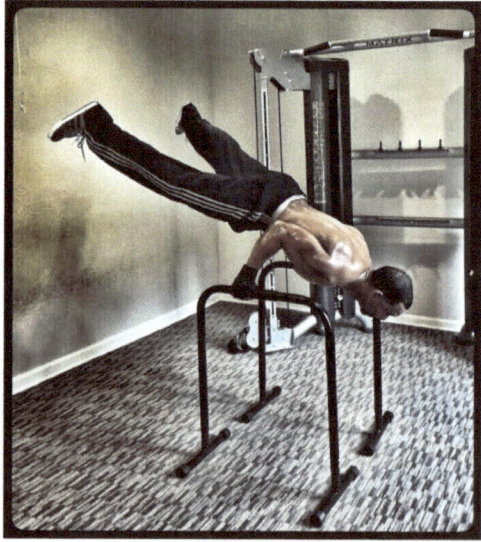

The Workouts

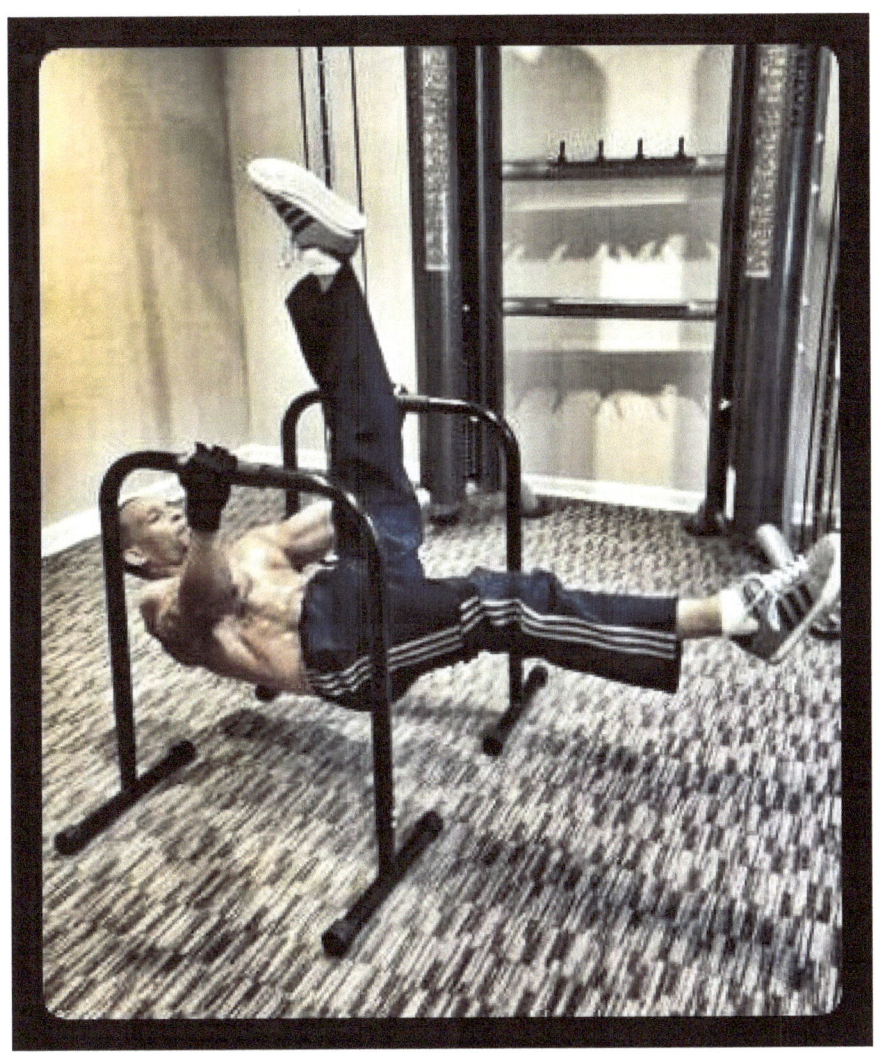

For Variation Numbers: Main Move (Dips), 2-12, 15-17, 19-23, 25, 27-29, 31, 39-40

Level 1   Level 2   Level 3
3 sets of 5-7 reps   4-5 sets of 8-10 reps   6-8 sets of 10+ reps

For Variation Numbers: 14, 18, 26, 30

Level 1   Level 2   Level 3
3 sets of 15-17 kicks   4-5 sets of 18-20 kicks   6-8 sets of 21-25 kicks

For Variation Numbers: 13, 24

Level 1   Level 2   Level 3
3 sets of 20-25 secs   4-5 sets of 25-30 secs   6-8 sets of 30+ secs

For Variation Numbers: 32-38

Level 1   Level 2   Level 3
3 sets of 5-7 secs   4-5 sets of 8-10 secs   6-8 sets of 10+ secs

Diet/Meal Plans

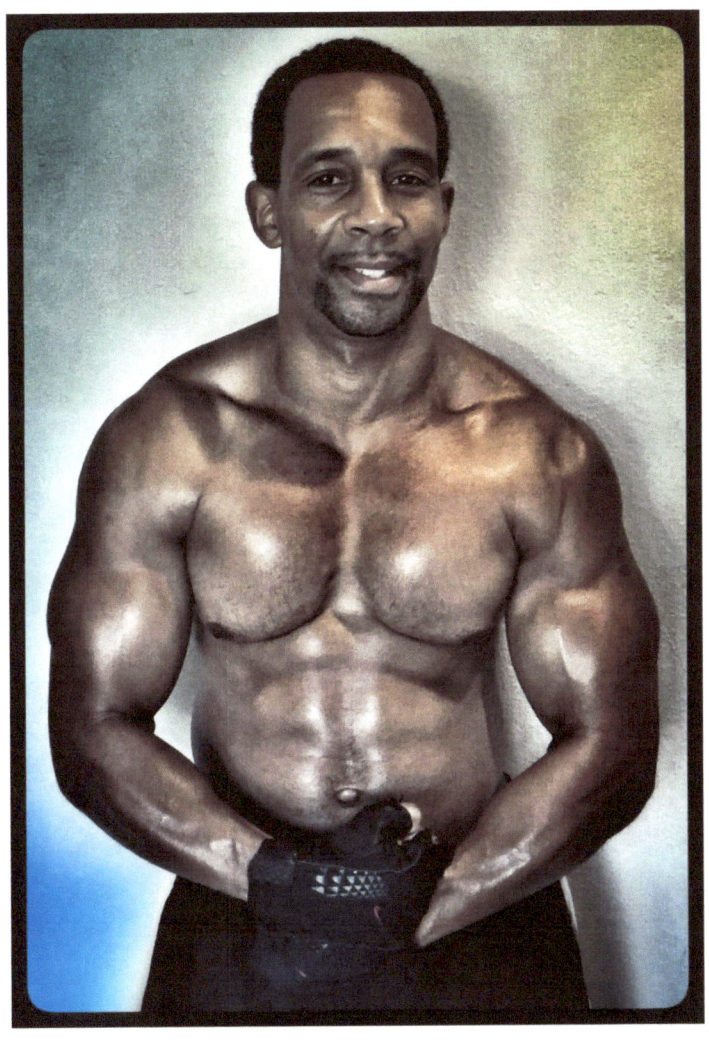

The Importance of Eating Healthy

To take your workout performance, physique, and attitude to the ultimate level, you must engage in a healthy nutritional diet plan. Believe it or not, if you want to have and lead a healthy lifestyle, good nutrition is at the top of the charts. You can really maximize your workouts and exercise results by simply putting the right foods in your body. In my early years of exercising, I didn't understand this concept and the importance of eating healthy. So while I was getting some results, I could never really go to the next level with my physique and strength. You see, the right foods will give you the energy, endurance, stamina and strength your body needs to maximize your results with your weekly workouts.

The right proteins will feed and repair your muscles post-workout. Salmon, chicken, and turkey are some of the many foods that provide a good source of protein for your muscles. Complex carbohydrates are the quickest source of energy because they are very rapidly digested. Energy is vital to any kind of workout! These foods consist of sweet potatoes, oatmeal, and whole grain breads, just to name a few.

I've composed a bonus weight gaining and weight loss diet plan depending on your health goals. Each diet consist of all natural foods that your body needs to stay healthy inside and out. The diet plans have the breakdown of each days' calories, proteins, and carbs for each meal. Right down to a "T", you'll know exactly what you're putting in your body.

As mentioned before, you can't maximize your results in the gym unless your diet is on point. Always remember, the best fashion statement is a healthy fit body...and the inside and out!

Low Calorie Diet

The Purpose of a Low Calorie Diet

The main focus of a low calorie diet is to promote healthy weight loss by restricting them from consuming foods that are simply high in calories. Let's use exercising as an example. If a person exercises regularly, they will burn more calories compared to the calories they consumed. When this takes place, the body then turns to the fats that's already stored to use it for energy purposes. This will eventually cause you to lose weight.

On average, most people consume about 2000-2500 calories a day. Most low calorie diets consist of 1500-1800 calories a day. In this book, I put together an effective and healthy 5-day a week low-calorie diet that will help you and your body go the extra mile to lose weight. My Monday-Friday meal plans will consist of less than 1500 calories per day.

Here are 6 benefits to eating a low calorie diet.

1. Weight loss
2. Helps cure health disease
3. Helps maintain weight management
4. Helps shred extra pounds
5. Speeds up metabolism
6. Burns fat

Low calorie diet proceeds on the following pages.

Brian Baker's 5-Day a Week Loss Diet – Under 1500 Calories per Day

Monday:

Breakfast
1 Bowl of Oatmeal with Skim Milk, 1 Slice of Whole Wheat Bread, and 2 Egg Whites
253 cal, 15.8g of protein, 39.4 carbs

Mid-Morning Snack
½ can of tuna and 1 cup of Greek yogurt
198.5 cal, 27.5g of protein, 15 carbs

Lunch
6-8 oz of grilled salmon and 1 cup of steamed broccoli
462 cal, 44.2g of protein, 10 carbs

Mid-Afternoon Snack
½ can of tuna and 1 cup of Greek yogurt
198.5 cal, 27.5g of protein, 15 carbs

Dinner
1 grilled chicken salad with 1 teaspoon of dressing and 1 cup of fresh grapes
331 cal, 40.6g of protein, 33 carbs

Total: 1,433 cal

Tuesday:

Breakfast
1 bowl of bran flake cereal w/ skim milk, 2 egg whites, 1 banana
259 cal, 12.2g of protein, 32.4 carbs

Mid-Morning Snack
½ an of tuna and 2 kiwi fruits
162.5 cal, 14.1g of protein, 20.2 carbs

Lunch
6-8 oz of broiled chicken breast and 1 cup of corn
297 cal, 29.1g of protein, 30.5 carbs

Mid-Afternoon Snack
½ can of tuna and 1 cup of pudding
418.5 cal, 21.5g of protein, 56 carbs

Dinner
6-8 oz of grilled tilapia, 1 cup of steamed broccoli, and 1 cup of sweet potatoes
276 cal, 29.3g of protein, 37 carbs

Total: 1,413 cal

Wednesday: Breakfast
1 bowl of shredded wheat cereal w/ skim milk, 1 slice of whole wheat bread, 2 egg whites
313 cal, 16.8g of protein, 52.4 carbs

Mid-Morning Snack
½ can of tuna and 1 cup of Greek yogurt
198.5 cal, 27.5g of protein, 15 carbs

Lunch
6-8 oz of roasted turkey breast w/o skin and 1 cup of green beans
184 cal, 35.8g of protein, 7 carbs

Mid-Afternoon Snack
½ can of tuna and 1 cup of Greek yogurt
198.5 cal, 27.5g of protein, 15 carbs

Dinner
6 oz of beef sirloin tip steak, 1 baked potato, 1 cup of cantaloupe
473 cal, 37.4g of protein, 49.5 carbs

Total: 1,367 cal

Thursday: Breakfast
1 Thomas 100% Whole Wheat Bagel, 2 egg whites, 1 cup of fresh blueberries
410 cal, 19.2g of protein, 82.7 carbs

Mid-Morning Snack
½ can of tuna and 1 serving of mozzarella sticks
208.5 cal, 18.5g of protein, 13 carbs

Lunch
6-8 oz of grilled flounder and 1 cup of steamed peas
172 cal, 23.6g of protein, 13.7 carbs

Mid-Afternoon Snack
½ can of tuna and 1 cup of cottage cheese
300.5 cal, 37.5g of protein, 8 carbs

Dinner
6-8 oz of baked chicken breast, 1 cup of brown rice, 1 small garden salad w/ 1 teaspoon of dressing
400 cal, 30.8g of protein, 50 carbs

Total (*Thurs*): 1,491 cal

Friday: Breakfast
1 bowl of multigrain Cheerios w/ skim milk, 2 boiled eggs, and 1 cup of fresh
strawberries
344 cal, 15.6g of protein, 37.1 carbs

Mid-Morning Snack
½ can of tuna and 1 cup of unsweetened applesauce
127.5 cal, 12.7g of protein, 12.7 carbs

Lunch
Chicken Caesar Salad and 1 cup of watermelon
320 cal, 39.9g of protein, 37 carbs

Mid-Afternoon Snack
½ can of tuna and 1 cup of sliced mangos
177.5 cal, 13.9g of protein, 25 carbs

Dinner
6-8 oz of grilled salmon, 1 cup of asparagus, 1 cup of diced pineapples
513 cal, 43.8g of protein, 24.6 carbs

Total: 1,482 cal

*Note: You must consume 1 gallon of distilled water a day and 4-8oz of Calcium fortified orange juice a
day.

Other Healthy Drinks	Seasonings	Other Healthy Snacks
Pomegranate Juice	Mrs. Dash	Protein Shakes
Low Fat Milk	Pepper	Protein Bars
Green Tea	Lemon Pepper	Tofu
Lemon Juice	Natural Dark Honey	Cinnamon Rice Cakes
Kale Juice	Cinnamon	Fresh Fruit & Veggies

High Calorie Diet

The Purpose of a High Calorie Diet

The main purpose of a high calorie diet is to help a person gain weight. But of course, it doesn't stop there. For a person who leads a very active and physically demanding lifestyle such as a professional athlete, a nutritionist or a doctor may prescribe a high calorie diet to fuel their bodies so they can achieve maximum results to improve their health. Usually people with fast or high metabolism should be recommended for a high calorie diet because their body burns fat at a faster rate. Therefore the weight they would gain would be quality weight and not just a bunch of fatty weight.

Most diets over 2500 calories are considered high calorie diets. In this book, I put together a healthy and effective 5-day a week high calorie diet plan. From Monday-Friday, each daily plan consist of a little over 3000 calories a day. Quality food combinations from this diet plan will cause your body to experience healthy changes in body composition.

Here are 6 benefits to eating a high calorie diet:

1. Helps with weight gain
2. Improves memory
3. Lowers blood pressure
4. Adds nutritional value to your body
5. Helps with skin, hair, and muscle repair
6. Boost energy

High calorie diet proceeds on the following pages.

Brian Baker's 5-Day a Week Weight Gain Diet – 3000+ Calories per Day

Monday:

Breakfast
3 whole wheat pancakes, 2 scrambled eggs, 1 cup of hash browns
928 cal, 25.3g of protein, 82.9 carbs

Mid-Morning Snack
1 cup of Greek yogurt, 1 tablespoon of peanut butter, 1 banana
319 cal, 20.3g of protein, 45 carbs

Lunch
1 Caesar salad with crispy chicken, 2 garlic bread slices, ½ slice mango
806.5 cal, 36g of protein, 97.5 carbs

Mid-Afternoon Snack
1 cup of cottage cheese
222 cal, 25g of protein, 8 carbs

Dinner
1 6oz of grilled salmon, 1 baked potato, 2 cups of corn, 1 slice of whole wheat bread
941 cal, 56.5g of protein, 109.5 carbs

Post-Dinner Snack
1 cup of sliced pineapple
74 cal, .84g of protein, 19.6 carbs

Total: 3,290 cal

Tuesday:

Breakfast
1 bowl of oatmeal w/ skim milk, 4 boiled eggs, 1 glass of cranberry juice
579 cal, 30g of protein, 60.4 carbs

Mid-Morning Snack
100g of trail mix
484 cal, 14g of protein, 45 carbs

Lunch
1 6oz of fillet mignon, ½ cup of pistachio nuts, 1 cup of steamed broccoli
849.5 cal, 60.7g of protein, 27 carbs

Mid-Afternoon Snack
1 fruit smoothie w/ whey protein powder
305 cal, 19.8g of protein, 17.3 carbs

Dinner
2 fillets of grilled tilapia, 2 tablespoons of garlic butter, 1 medium side portion of red potatoes, 2 cups of green beans
640 cal, 53.8g of protein, 48.2 carbs

Post-Dinner Snack
1 cup of sliced avocado
234 cal, 2.9g of protein, 12 carbs

Total: 3,091 cal

Wednesday: Breakfast
2 whole wheat waffles, 2 large egg cheese omelets, 1 cinnamon raisin bagel, 1 cup of mangos
745 cal, 29.2g of protein, 84.7 carbs

Mid-Morning Snack
1 protein bar
331 cal, 20g of protein, 40 carbs

Lunch
1 8oz ribeye steak cooked in a tablespoon of oil, 1 cup of sweet potatoes, and 1 pear
750 cal, 72.1g of protein, 50 carbs

Mid-Afternoon Snack
1oz of mixed nuts
175 cal, 4.7g of protein, 6.1 carbs

Dinner
1 serving size of grilled tuna steak, 1 baked potato w/ garlic butter, 2 cups of corn
818 cal, 65.8g of protein, 97.9 carbs

Post-Dinner Snack
1 red white and blue cottage cheese fruit salad
195 cal, 12g of protein, 26.6 carbs

Total: 3,014 cal

Thursday: Breakfast
1 steak and cheese omelet, 1 cup of strawberries, 2 slices of whole wheat butter toast, 1 8oz glass of O.J
745.6 cal, 44.2g of protein, 66 carbs

Mid-Morning Snack
1 mango pineapple smoothie
326 cal, 4g of protein, 64 carbs

Lunch
1 ½ fillet grilled halibut, 1 cup of brown rice, 2 whole wheat pita breads
935 cal, 46g of protein, 115 carbs

Mid-Afternoon Snack
½ can of tuna and 1 cup of Greek yogurt
198.5 cal, 27.5g of protein, 15 carbs

Dinner
1 8oz serving of lean beef brisket, 1 cup of whole wheat macaroni, 1 cup of green soy beans
544.9 cal, 104.5g of protein, 65.2 carbs

Post-Dinner Snack
1 cup of figs
279 cal, 1g of protein, 73 carbs

Total: 3,422.1 cal

Friday: Breakfast
3 slices of French toast with 2% milk, 2 scrambled eggs w/ cheese, 2 slices of turkey bacon, 1 8oz glass of low-fat milk
873 cal, 45g of protein, 64 carbs

Mid-Morning Snack
½ cup of raisins, seedless
217 cal, 2.2g of protein, 57.5 carbs

Lunch
1 grilled chicken sandwich, 1 serving of homemade French fries (1 potato), 1 cup of grapes
500 cal, 32.6g of protein, 87 carbs

Mid-Afternoon Snack
1 16oz strawberry banana smooth w/ whey protein
313 cal, 30g of protein, 43 carbs

Dinner
2 fillets of sea bass, 1 baked potato w/ butter and sour cream, 1 cup of sweet corn,
2 slices of butter wheat toast
869 cal, 65.2g of protein, 103.6 carbs

Post-Dinner Snack
2oz of cashew nuts
314 cal, 10g of protein, 18 carbs

Total: 3,086 cal

*Note: You must consume 1 gallon of distilled water a day and 4-8oz of Calcium fortified orange juice a day.

Other Healthy Drinks	Seasonings	Other Healthy Snacks
Pomegranate Juice	Mrs. Dash	Protein Shakes
Low Fat Milk	Pepper	Protein Bars
Green Tea	Lemon Pepper	Tofu
Lemon Juice	Natural Dark Honey	Cinnamon Rice Cakes
Kale Juice	Cinnamon	Fresh Fruit & Veggies

Conclusion

Throughout this book I've shared with you the importance and effectiveness of the parallel bars. From the advantages, various exercises, and health tips, the parallel bars are a win-win situation for your workout program. I've been working with these bars for 10+ years and they've truly taken my health and strength to a whole new level.

Being a personal trainer for over 15 years now, I understand that body weight exercises and versatility to your workout program is crucial for seeing the amazing results that you deserve. By incorporating the variations to your weekly workout routine, not only will you get stronger in body weight exercises, but also stronger in performing weight lifting exercises. In addition to, your cardiovascular routines will improve dramatically as well.

For maximum results, it's wise to change up your workout regimen every 10-14 days. With these 40 different variations of parallel bar exercises, you will be able to constantly shock your muscles into the type of physique that you've always dreamed of. I hope and pray that this book becomes a blessing to you.

God Bless!

The Cobra Back

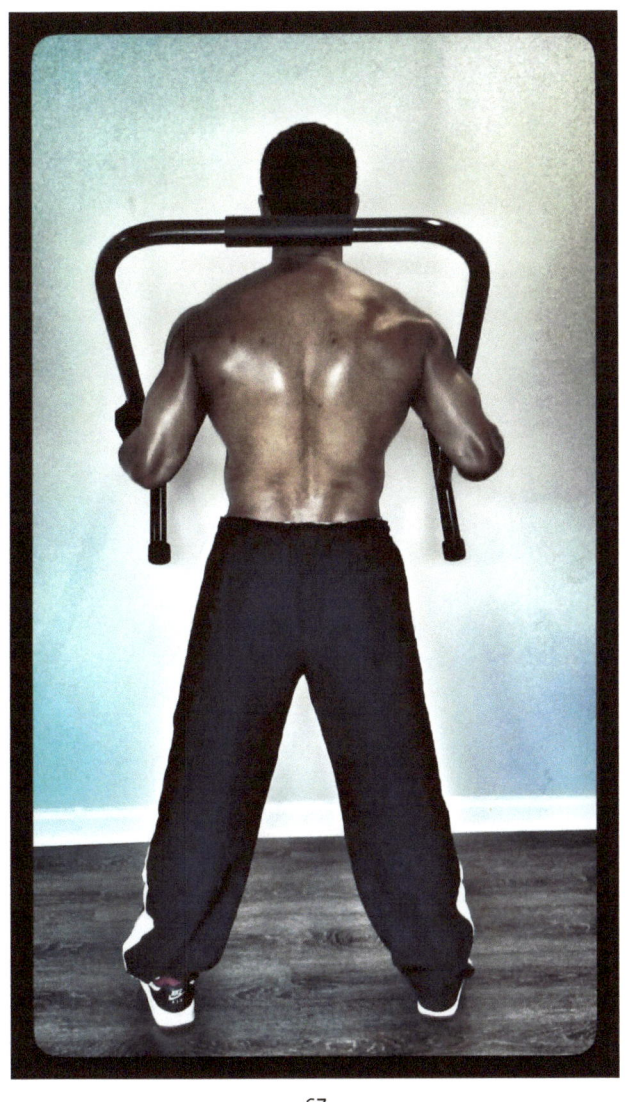